MEMOIRS OF A SURGEON'S WIFE:

I'm Throwing Your Damn Pager into the Ocean

By Megan Sharma

Copyright 2018 Megan Sharma
Print Edition
All rights reserved

Memoirs of a Surgeon's Wife, by Megan Sharma

COPYRIGHT INFORMATION

No part of this publication may be reproduced, distributed, or transmitted in any form by any means, including photocopying, recording, or other electronic or mechanical methods, without the prior written permission of the publisher, except in the case of brief quotations embodied in reviews and certain other non-commercial uses permitted by copyright law.

Contact the publisher at www.megansharma.com, or email megan@megansharma.com.

Memoirs of a Surgeon's Wife, by Megan Sharma

DEDICATION

For my incredible husband, Arun, who has always been my biggest supporter, and for our indomitable daughter, Jasmine. You two are my everything.

♦ ♦ ♦

"There is only one happiness in this life, to love and be loved." –George Sand

Memoirs of a Surgeon's Wife, by Megan Sharma

TABLE OF CONTENTS

Copyright information..3
Dedication..5
Foreword..9
Part 1: Let's make small talk...13
Part 2: Our love story...29
Part 3: Life in the trenches: residency..55
Part 4: Life beyond residency..211
The back of book stuff..239
References..253

Memoirs of a Surgeon's Wife, by Megan Sharma

FOREWORD

About two years ago, shortly after I first met Megan and Arun Sharma, Megan asked me to read and critique the initial manuscript of her as-yet-unpublished book. She reasoned that since, like her, I am a writer, and, like her husband, Arun, I am also a physician, I could offer her some helpful advice. She told me that the premise of her book— well described by its engaging title— was a combination of personal memoir and survival guide for spouses of physicians, especially of physicians still in school or in residency/fellowship training.

What Megan did not tell me was that she is a superb writer, possessed of total command of the English language, including her ability to deliver in prose her phenomenal sense of wit and understated humor (she should have also warned me that my hernia would be at risk from laughing so hard and so often.) Furthermore, she did not mention the extraordinary amount of research she had done to cover so thoroughly the myriad entities and challenges that confront spouses of physicians.

And so, I proceeded to read with great pleasure that initial manuscript. I advised Megan that in all my years in medicine I had never come across a book quite like it in scope and that she should confidently get on with the process to publish it. I came up with nothing to criticize about the book's content, but Megan still had a few ideas to expand upon the book to make it even better.

When Megan invited me to write the foreword for the final manuscript of the book (or e-reader) that you now hold in your hands, I readily agreed to the honor, concurrently thinking to myself: "Should be really easy to do this for a book that I think is terrific." Well, folks, it has not been that easy, because "Memoirs of a Surgeon's Wife" covers so much territory.

Memoirs of a Surgeon's Wife, by Megan Sharma

To start, we have a love story— beautifully told, with much interspersed humor and whimsy— of a talented couple from vastly different backgrounds. We can never get too much of these types of stories, right? Megan and Arun, along with their lovely young daughter, Jasmine, are a joy to get to know.

Then we move on to the challenges of marriage to a spouse consumed by professional commitments, with all the attendant exigencies and deprivations, day after day, year after year. As Megan reminds us, the interminable on-call way of life can really wear you down. As a physician who went through it, myself, for so many years, I believe that it is THE most difficult thing to handle for a physician and his or her family. Thus, the importance of Megan's expansive and detailed section on "Life in the Trenches: Residency." For some, reading this section might literally be marriage-saving, and perhaps even life-saving. This subject correctly occupies the largest portion of the book.

One of my favorite chapters is the one titled "Bad Ass Women in Medicine." Mercifully, sufficient social enlightenment has occurred to give us optimism that chauvinism and sexism are finally on the way out, but these despicable attitudes were certainly the order of the day in the times of these courageous women who overcame prodigious obstacles to become superior physicians. I consider this segment to be the gem of the book's many delightful digressions.

While this is a book that will entertain and expand the horizons of readers from all walks of life, I say that it should be required reading for all medical students, physicians, their spouses, and prospective spouses, who find themselves in the challenging years of medical training. Also, those who contemplate to enter the medical profession should consider Megan's book to be a pre-med, pre-marriage requirement.

"...and just one more thing," as my favorite TV character, Columbo, would say. So, what's up with that funky subtitle, "I'm Throwing Your Damn Pager into the Ocean"? For thirty years, 1976 through 2006, I carried a pager (a beeper, as I called it), pretty much 24/7, except occasionally while on vacation. I always wore it on the left side of my belt, above my left hip, and always in the vibration mode. For those 30 years, about ten times a day I would feel the vibrations of the pager— disrupting, anxiety-provoking, calling me to immediate attention. Then in 2006, I converted from the pager to a cell phone which included the pager function. No more vibrations on the left side of my belly. Except, NO! Not the case at all. Those vibrations—phantom vibrations— exactly where I used to carry my beeper, still occurred several times a day; constant reminders of the on-call life. Over the years

Memoirs of a Surgeon's Wife, by Megan Sharma

the frequency of these phantom vibrations has decreased, but I still get them to this day, perhaps once a week. They are an atavistic nuisance. I really would like to get rid of them.

I, therefore, take the liberty here to petition Megan Sharma: "Please also throw MY damn phantom pager into the ocean."

Now go forth and enjoy this terrific book.

Eli Goodman, M.D.
www.eligoodmanmd.com
Springfield, Illinois
June 2018

Memoirs of a Surgeon's Wife, by Megan Sharma

PART 1: LET'S MAKE SMALL TALK

❖ ❖ ❖ ❖ ❖

Memoirs of a Surgeon's Wife, by Megan Sharma

BACK TO THE FUTURE

Half of my worldly belongings are covered in green, recyclable bubble wrap. The other half are shoved hastily into a box and then excessively taped or sheltered by a heavy gray moving blanket with hopes of avoiding damage during the cross-country journey from Seattle to Pittsburgh.

We're almost to the finish line, and yet, I feel like I'm taking several steps backward. My husband and I are getting ready to move in with my parents—and I'm over 30. I'm preparing to leave behind the hometown I have loved since my early teens, along with all my friends and my immediate family.

I am also pregnant, a joy which I won't know until shortly after moving back in with my parents.

Congratulations are in order. We are taking the next step.

Will it be worth the sacrifice?

Our baby will be born in a strange city where people commonly eat fries on green salad. We won't have our strong network surrounding us, as we did in the Pacific Northwest.

We'll see how I feel on residency graduation day...

Memoirs of a Surgeon's Wife, by Megan Sharma

IS THIS BOOK FOR ME?

It's important to consider the commitment involved in reading anything longer than 280 characters. How will you know if this book is for you? Are we reader/author soul mates? Take this easy quiz to find out!

- ☐ Have you ever been royally bitch slapped by a fortune cookie ("Your exercise routine needs improvement")?
- ☐ When you turned 18, did you immediately go with all your friends to get a belly button ring, tattoo, or nose piercing?
- ☐ Did you rock out to Destiny's Child, Backstreet Boys, and *NSYNC as a teenager?
- ☐ Do you find strange glee in discovering grammar and usage errors on menus at Vietnamese restaurants, on billboards and in advertorials?
- ☐ Have you ever stubbed your toe so hard that it bruised underneath the nail, while you were doing nothing but attempting to walk through a door?
- ☐ When you're feeling frisky, do you eat brownies for breakfast, and then let your Facebook friends know you've done so, by way of confession?
- ☐ Is H_2O your favorite compound?
- ☐ Are you enamored of Victorian architecture and harmonious prose?
- ☐ Do you never, ever want to be involved with climbing Everest?
- ☐ Would your friends describe you as "the one who always makes the birthday cake"?
- ☐ Is your living room floor littered with magnetic blocks, little wooden musical instruments, baby teethers, board books, rainbow stacking cups, soft edged kitchen tools, and every single throw pillow from all three of your couches?
- ☐ Do you tend to forget things unless you write them down? (Note to self: refill prescription!)

Memoirs of a Surgeon's Wife, by Megan Sharma

If you answered yes to at least half of these questions, CONGRATULATIONS! It doesn't make any difference whatsoever. I just wanted to see if we had anything in common. But you should definitely read this book, no matter what your answers were!

Memoirs of a Surgeon's Wife, by Megan Sharma

HELLO! LET'S GET ACQUAINTED

My name is Megan. I'm just a Millennial girl who fell in love with and married a doctor. A surgeon, to be precise. Of course, growing up in America, I've seen my fair share of romantic comedies and TV shows featuring alluring doctor heroes with impeccable pearly whites, like "The Wedding Planner" and "Scrubs." Yet, I never targeted getting hitched to an M.D. as one of my life goals. It just wasn't on the radar. That is, until I met my husband, Arun. But I'll tell you more about that in due time. First, please indulge me ever so briefly, and I'll give you a little background on me and how I came to write this book.

I've been writing since I was a little kid circa age 10, when there was no such thing as a tween and the only computer font available was neon green on a black screen. It's been a near lifelong infatuation, so I am especially psyched out of my mind to have published this book. I am doing rock star scissor kicks while wearing snakeskin pants in my imagination at this very moment.

I have a natural sense of curiosity which was further magnified and honed by my education in journalism. As such, you will notice that this book contains many different tones and topics related to life on the inside of modern medicine. While reading, you should expect to chuckle one minute and gather all your righteous indignation for a serious topic the next.

At some point in my career, which has ranged from government and politics to corporate marketing and communications, I decided, you know what? I don't want to write almost exclusively in acronyms anymore. I don't care about how

Memoirs of a Surgeon's Wife, by Megan Sharma

best to position some slippery technology concept. Let's go ahead and broaden that horizon—I want to write about what I want to write about.

Great. Certainly admirable. But, where to start?

Well, I don't know enough about vampires or wizards to make a name for myself (darn you, Stephenie Meyer and J. K. Rowling! You have a monopoly!) I know some. Not enough for a book deal.

What I am intimately familiar with, big shocker here, is my own life. And my life involves the life of my husband, who is a surgeon, and our life together as a married couple.

Over the years, we've laughed, cried, cringed, and told shocking stories to all our friends and family. One day in October 2013 I literally woke up feeling inspired (how rare and wonderful is that?) and decided, why not share our story with the world, so that you, too, can have a good belly laugh, and then make a mental note to ask your surgeon if they've been sleeping enough lately.

Memoirs of a Surgeon's Wife, by Megan Sharma

GREAT EXPECTATIONS

Expectations are the super-secret key that unlocks either our happiness, satisfaction and glee or our disappointment, disillusionment and sour pucker face. Any qualified therapist will tell you this, however more eloquently, and with a far heftier price tag.

With that in mind, I want to be clear about what this book is, and why it exists. This is not a tell-all: it's a tell *most*. There are certain subjects that I do not touch with a ten-foot pole because I believe they are extremely personal. These topics include sex, religion, and detailed accounts of marital discord featuring all the most incendiary he said, she said moments.

Think about it. Would *you* want to reveal the details of your sex life to your mother, your in-laws, and your husband's esteemed colleagues? I'd venture to say that most of us wouldn't. Not all of us are as ballsy as Chelsea Handler (go, girl!).

Now, as to why this book exists. In a word: love. I wrote this book out of love and a desire to share our experiences. So, if you're looking for a book that villainizes the workaholic surgeon husband and details the minutiae of his wrongdoing, look elsewhere.

If you're ready for a love story set against the backdrop of modern medicine, read on, my friends. Read on.

Memoirs of a Surgeon's Wife, by Megan Sharma

MUSINGS FROM MY 11-YEAR-OLD SELF

"In the future, I predict that a lot of changes will take place in my life. I might have completely different interests, feelings, opinions, and values. Of course, no one can tell the future, but I know that these different views might enter my mind. Even though I might have some of the same friends, I'm going to be very different from the eleven-year-old girl I am today."

I am quoting myself. At age 11. WHAT??

I have my teachers to thank for that. I recently unearthed not one, but three autobiographical works by yours truly. What better way to get to know me than to delve into the workings of my adolescent brain?

Here is an excerpt from a chapter of my 6th grade autobiography, titled: "My Future Dreams." I'm typing it exactly as it's written on paper, since that is half the charm. This was clearly before spell check was invented. I believe it was typed on my mom's old typewriter. That automatically gives me street cred, right? I will also add [*the reality of what happened*] in italicized brackets, 20 years later.

High School Shenanigans
"Here's how I see it. Megan Marsh [*my maiden name*], student at Lynbrook High School [*this was the high school I would have attended, had my family not moved from San Jose, California to Federal Way, Washington two years later*], getting all A's [*I got close to all A's and took AP classes. GPA was 3.75*], yet nervous about college [*I only applied to one school and I wasn't nervous about it. I got in*]. Yea, it's true, but there's alot more to it than that. In my high school years, I see myself as a cheerleader who can

Memoirs of a Surgeon's Wife, by Megan Sharma

still keep up her grades [*that's exactly what happened! I cheered for three years*]. Sure, I don't exactly look like a cheerleader now [*I was chubby*], but there is a lot of time ahead of me before my Lynbrook years [*I lost weight the next year*]. Besides being involved with sports, I think that I will want to join a few clubs. I'm interested in choir, band, and drama club [*I joined none of these clubs*]. Of course you probably ask how can I possibly keep my grades up, and also be involved with all of these time consuming activities. Well, right now, I even play an instrument [*the piano, which I hated and only played for two years*], and I do fantastic in school. Whew! I guess that about sums it up for high school." [*apparently finishing that summary was a great weight off my shoulders*]

College
"Well, now that I've graduated high school, I'm off to....hmmmmm....Point Loma Nazerine College....or Berkeley? Oh, which one should I choose [*I chose Seattle Pacific University in Washington state*]? Let's see, Point Loma is closer and has better surroundings, but Berkeley is more challenging! Alright, I've made up my mind, I choose Point Loma. It has people of my own Christian faith, and I'll probably never have to face the temptation of drinking, smoking, or doing drugs [*hilarious!*]. Horray for me! Choosing a college is a very important decision. It decides what you will major in, and what kind of job you will get [*Ummm...no. Not so much*]. Right now, I want to have my name in the theatre, and I hope to be a star [*I don't even remember wanting to be in show business! I think I had performed in a few church plays at this point*]. But if I don't make it into show business [*didn't happen, didn't try*], I hope to be a singer [*nope*] or an artist [*I still consider myself an artist. I paint, write and take photos in my spare time*]. With this in mind, I think I will major in Graphic Designing [*great! "Graphic Designing", a major that doesn't even exist! I majored in journalism.*]."

Finding Mr. Right
"After four long years of college, I am finally ready to get out into the real world [*the real world is much scarier!*]. I am not going to get married until I find ' Mr. Right ' [*so glad this really happened*]. After he is found, I am going to get married, but wait to start a family. If I had children too soon, I might not be ready financially to start a career, and be a mother at the same time [*good lord, how was I so wise?*]. I'd have the responsibility to nurse and care for a human being, and I don't think that I will be ready for that the first year of marrage [*we had our first child 2.5 years after our wedding*]. However, once I get my career going, being a cartoonist [*WTF????*], I might be ready to have children [*because cartooning and procreation obviously go hand in hand*]. I would live with my husband in Monterey, California, right by the ocean [*we currently live in the middle of Illinois. There is no ocean here*]. This would be great because we could stroll along the beaches, and if we had children, they'd have tons of fun on

Memoirs of a Surgeon's Wife, by Megan Sharma

the wharf and making sandcastles [*our daughter loves the beach!*]. I'd like the weather always in the 70's" [*wouldn't we all?*].

My Life as a Married Woman

"I think that I'd have a schedule for each day. Say, first, I get up, brush my teeth, shower, and dress [*groundbreaking stuff*]. Next, I'll make breakfast, and take the kids to school. Then, at about 9:00, I'll go to work. I'll come home at about 6:00, and make dinner. At 6:30, I'll call the kids in, and we'll have a nice family meal [*sounds wonderful, mini June Cleaver!*]. After dinner, the kids will do their homework, and I'll relax [*guess I won't be helping them with said homework*]. At 10:00, I'll go to bed, and get up at 7:00 the next morning. In my free time, I, Megan _____ [*Sharma*], will probably enjoy cooking and sewing [*the only thing I've ever sewn is a bandana. But I love cooking*]. If my husband really loves me, he'll watch the kids when I'm exhausted [*yes on both accounts*].

When 30 Happens

"By the year 2013, I will be 30 years old. YIKES! I could never see myself being that old, but it has to happen sometime [*truth. And I'm now over 30*]. Well, anyway, when I'm 30, I think that the medical world will be A LOT more advanced. Doctors might even find a cure for cancer, and AIDS [*still working on both efforts*]. It would save millions of lifes if they did. I think that the world will have long completed, and perfected the solar car [*I was right about one thing, strangely enough*]. Then we would have a less polluted world, and a better environment for plants and animals [*if only*].

◆ ◆ ◆

Well, that's enough humiliation for now. Hope you enjoyed that magical journey through my pre-teen mind.

Memoirs of a Surgeon's Wife, by Megan Sharma

MY BRAND OF FEMINISM

You will notice a theme in this book: I am a proud feminist, and I'm passionate about gender equity. Since everyone defines feminism differently, let me explain what it means to me.

My feminist credo:

- I believe in equity for all people and opportunity for all to shine.
- We all have our conscious or unconscious personal biases. The key to a better world is to be aware of these biases and to think about how they may impact how we treat others.
- I believe in the power of choice. Empowering women means empowering their choices. As a stay-at-home mom, a full-time corporate powerhouse, an entrepreneur, or something of your own design—you can lean in however you want to. Yes, I have read "Lean In." I am trying to lean in right now by writing this book!
- Women should be able to follow their dreams and become their own bosses, if they so desire.
- We still have more work to do. Like, a LOT more work to do. Boatloads. There are systems in place that make it more difficult for women to succeed, and we are definitely not equal. In the 21st century, why do we still have a pay gap between men and women who are doing the exact same work? It's unjustifiable and we need to act.
- While both my husband and I were raised in households with fairly traditional gender roles, we believe that a husband and wife are partners and equals. I do dishes, laundry and child care and so does my husband. We do whatever it takes to keep our household running smoothly as a team.

Memoirs of a Surgeon's Wife, by Megan Sharma

- Partnership doesn't always mean precisely 50/50. Yes, I tend to cook more often and spend more time caring for our daughter. My husband also works 60-70 hours per week. We don't get caught up in the math.
- Some things are a matter of personal preference, like taking your husband's name. I will be perfectly honest. I didn't want to give up my maiden name. It's so weird to relinquish a name you've had your entire life. Am I right, ladies? But I also wanted to unite our family and future children by sharing the same family name.
- Women should pursue any field or endeavor they are passionate about. I want that for my daughter and for every young girl from Boston to Botswana.
- I shouldn't be looked down on because I am a take-charge kind of person who happens to be a woman. That doesn't make me bossy.

Now you know where I'm coming from, boys and girls.

"A woman is like a tea bag - you can't tell how strong she is until you put her in hot water." –Eleanor Roosevelt

Memoirs of a Surgeon's Wife, by Megan Sharma

PART 2: OUR LOVE STORY

❖ ❖ ❖ ❖ ❖

Memoirs of a Surgeon's Wife, by Megan Sharma

EARLY DAYS: HOW WE MET AND FELL IN LOVE

Let me set the scene. My husband and I met in the emerald city, Seattle. They call it the emerald city because of its lush greenery—one benefit of the ever-present rain. Until we moved away in 2014, the iconic Space Needle was literally in our backyard (and by backyard, I mean a short series of alleys, city streets and pay-per-hour parking lots).

Seattle is the land of $7 triple grande soy lattes, an abundance of tech companies, booming real estate, and recycled toilet paper. Yes, people buy recycled toilet paper in this city. I am not one of those people. The mere thought of recycled toilet paper is mildly repulsive and prevents me from even a perfunctory Google search on the actual process of creating such an environmentally-friendly product. Maybe you can do it for me and Tweet at me with the results.

Okay, set the clock back to December 2008. Many Seattleites remember the last couple of weeks of that year as the blizzard of 2008, during which record snow fell and the city completely shut down, ill-equipped to handle anything more than a dusting, especially with the steeply graded, narrow city streets characteristic of the metropolitan area.

At the time, I owned a 2004 Chrysler PT Cruiser, candy apple red with chrome accents and tinted windows. Totally pimped. It was fondly dubbed the PT Loser by my friends and lived up to the name because it couldn't even power over a slight drift in the driveway. So, I wasn't going anywhere until the snow cleared up. Thankfully I was on a two-week vacation for the holidays, anyway.

Memoirs of a Surgeon's Wife, by Megan Sharma

What to do with so much idle time and Christmas shopping a faraway memory? Shop for a boyfriend on Match.com, of course! I was 25 and ready to meet someone with long-term potential.

This was before the era of Tinder (thank heavens!) If I had been subjected to Tinder, I probably would have opted to become a nun. The Tinder conversations my friends pass along are simply appalling. I can't repeat them here.

At least Match.com is a paid service and therefore weeds out a portion of the riff raff. After receiving a wink (a noncommittal form of online flirting) from an attractive, normal-looking guy named Arun who listed watching "Lost" and cooking as hobbies on his online profile, we exchanged several emails. At first, I thought it was odd and slightly suspicious that many of his emails came in after 1:00 a.m., but then he explained that he was currently working the night shift on his emergency department rotation, from 7:00 p.m. to 7:00 a.m., with occasional down time in the middle of the night.

Finally, just as I was starting to get a little looney from too much time in close quarters with my equally punchy roommates, Arun proposed that we meet for coffee at Herkimer in the Greenwood neighborhood of Seattle, just a few miles from where I was living.

We met on the eve of New Year's Eve, December 30th, at the coffee shop. We arrived and were crossing the street at the same time, so we walked in together. We were greeted to the charged silence of one of those über serious studying/work only cafes. No chatter allowed. I knew immediately that we had to get out of there. There was no way in HELL I was going to share my first date, with all implicit first date awkwardness, with a room full of judgmental hipsters. Nah-uh.

I suggested that we take our java to go and hit the sidewalk for a neighborhood sip and stroll.

At the time, it was the height of the economic depression and Greenwood Avenue North was indeed a bit depressing, filled with the ghosts of small business' past. I tried to point out interesting landmarks: "That used to be a beauty school. I never went there." "This place has the best hot chocolate. And fortune cookies with naughty fortunes." And "My friend Jill lives in that tiny apartment there!" I am quite the conversational acrobat, as you can see.

Memoirs of a Surgeon's Wife, by Megan Sharma

Arun was quiet. I mean, exceptionally mum. It wasn't rude, he just seemed to be listening and taking it all in. Listening. How confusing. What was this alien dating behavior?

Before we met I knew that Arun had just started his surgical residency a few months prior, and that he was a doctor. I was a little worried about topics of conversation and if he would think I was a dummy, especially because the only vague ideas I had about a residency program were gleaned from "Grey's Anatomy". Not the best source for credible medical field intelligence. But that McDreamy, though... I digress.

The fact that Arun wasn't saying much on our date put me into nervous Chatty Kathie overdrive, and I barely paused for breath over the course of what turned out to be nearly a two-mile walk.

When we arrived back at Herkimer, I was pleasantly surprised to witness some traditional manners when Arun offered to walk me to my car (in a non-creepy way) and gave me a big hug. He said he enjoyed our time and we parted ways.

I left the date feeling slightly befuddled. I had indeed enjoyed the date, but Arun had barely said three words to me! Did he have a jolly good time? I figured that I would know soon enough by the follow up or lack thereof: where the rubber meets the road.

I got my answer the following evening on New Year's Eve. I was third-wheeling a sushi feast with my married friends Chad and Kiara when I got a phone call. To avoid obnoxiously talking on my phone at the restaurant, I let the call go to voicemail.

A few minutes later I checked the voicemail.

"You guys, it's the guy I went on a date with yesterday," I said. Obviously, I had told them all about the date already. "OOOOoohhh!" they replied in ill-concealed glee. "He asked me out on another date over voicemail. What do I do?" "Call him back!!!" they screamed.

I decided to wait to call him back until after dinner. Unfortunately, he was already knee deep in NYE disasters by that time (he had the good fortune of taking call that night) and we didn't connect until the following day, except for the "Happy New Year!" text I sent at midnight.

Memoirs of a Surgeon's Wife, by Megan Sharma

On New Year's Day, we chatted and made plans for a second date. We would meet downtown, do lunch and check out the view from the Columbia Tower, the tallest skyscraper in Seattle and the entire state of Washington, rising 967 feet over 76 floors. (Yup, I looked it up).

I was impressed by this plan. First, it was a creative date idea. More importantly, it made me realize that Arun was a skilled and astute listener: I had mentioned that the view from the Columbia Tower was purportedly better than that of the Space Needle on our first date. He ran with that.

On our second date, we did more walking and more talking, but this time I got to learn more about Arun: his job, his family, and his former city of Pittsburgh. It was nice to hear his voice. And it prevented me from going hoarse, which I appreciated.

Arun had planned for lunch at a dim sum restaurant near the Columbia Tower. I had never tried dim sum, so I was excited. We entered O'Asian Kitchen, a cavernous, nightclub-esque establishment, and were seated quickly in a room empty of diners. Arun excused himself to use the restroom just after we were shown to our table.

During those few moments of his absence, a kind Asian woman came by wearing a broad smile and pushing a large cart full of unfamiliar delicacies. Without prelude, she asked me if I wanted shrimp balls. "Sure," I replied. How else should one reply to a question like that? "Dumplings?" "Yes, please." "Egg roll?" "Ummm...ok." By the time I realized what was happening, I had ordered our entire lunch while my date was in the bathroom.

"Oh, CRAP!" I thought to myself. "He is going to think I'm nuts!" I put on my brightest I'm-not-crazy grin as Arun returned to the table.

"Sooooo...I accidentally may have ordered our entire lunch while you were gone." To my great relief, he laughed it off. It wasn't a big deal. Thank you, Jesus!

After lunch, we enjoyed the incredible view from the Columbia Tower (watch out, Space Needle!), and made our way back uptown.

At the end of the date, after talking a bunch and ignoring several episodes of "Chappelle's Show," we shared our first kiss, and it was really something! I was

Memoirs of a Surgeon's Wife, by Megan Sharma

honestly surprised that someone so well-mannered and smart could give me that butterfly kind of feeling. I was giddy.

After our second date, we melted into that early dating stupor when all you want to do is spend time with the other person. We watched movies on Netflix, made out on the couch, and ate a LOT of chicken phad thai and phad kee mao. We both gained at least five pounds, but neither of us cared.

At some point my friends demanded to meet this guy who was occupying all my free time. We staged a few double dates and bar-side meet and greets. My friends were fascinated by the fact that I was dating a surgeon, someone who actually cuts people open for a living, as was I.

My friend Mike started calling Arun "the Surgeon General." At some point, we earned our own Brangelina (RIP!) status and we became the Marsharmas, a combination of our last names: Marsh and Sharma.

But we officially came out as a couple on Valentine's Day 2009, when friends Chad and Kiara threw a swanky cocktail party at their apartment building in upscale Mercer Island.

I will always remember that Valentine's Day for two reasons: 1) it was my first Valentine's Day with Arun and he had very thoughtfully surprised me by sending flowers (and swearing my roommates to secrecy until I could get home to see them), and by giving me a box of chocolates. This was no ordinary box of Godiva. Oh, no. At first inspection, I wondered why the chocolates were wrapped in aluminum foil. Aren't they normally just ready to eat? When I opened one, I realized that there was a tiny strip of paper inside each morsel with neat handwriting that said something about why Arun liked me, including "You make me laugh even when you are making fun of me."

Every single chocolate had a unique paper sentiment inside. How clever and sweet is that?

The second reason I will always remember that Valentine's Day is due to a blush-worthy exchange at the cocktail party. Kiara's mom, Jane (who is so much like my own mom it's freaky), was thrilled to meet Arun. Unbeknownst to Arun, Jane had already heard all about him, mostly secondhand from Kiara.

Memoirs of a Surgeon's Wife, by Megan Sharma

Jane's first question to Arun was this: "Now, you aren't going to take our Megan away from Seattle, are you?" Poor Arun was caught off guard. He took it in stride and said something to the effect of, "Not planning to any time soon!" We all still laugh about it to this day. Especially because Jane totally called that one!

Even in the early days of our relationship, I knew that it was different. I explained it to my girlfriends like this: "I never had to wonder if he liked me."

Sounds like a small thing, but in the unforgiving wilderness of the dating world, it is hugely significant not to deal with games like fragmented calling patterns and even flirting with other girls right in front of you.

I was happy. And he treated me well. And, we soon discovered, we were falling in love.

Memoirs of a Surgeon's Wife, by Megan Sharma

THE L WORD

I remember clearly the exact moment Arun dropped the L word on me: Love. After three whole months of dating. We had attended a large group birthday party that evening and were snuggling back at home. "Honey..." he said, his pause dripping with meaning.

I waited with bated breath.

Perhaps it was because my own feelings were so strong, but I knew exactly what he was about to say.

"I love you."

It was such a relief to hear because my heart was screaming the same and I could finally say the words. "I love you, too!"

I confessed that I had wanted to tell him the same but had waited to hear it from him first to make sure it was real and mutual.

Ever since, we are like broken records on this topic. We probably say "I love you" at least 27 times every day. It's one of those habits that we can't break and have no desire to. We're lucky that way.

Memoirs of a Surgeon's Wife, by Megan Sharma

THE ENGAGEMENT THAT ALMOST WASN'T

Our engagement almost didn't happen. Snow conspired to keep us apart, but in the end, it was Arun and Megan-1, Mother Nature-0.

It was December 2010. I had flown to Northern California to surprise my grandparents and extended family on Christmas day, while Arun had spent the holidays with his family outside of Philadelphia. A tale of two coasts.

We had planned to reunite before New Year's for a mini-vacation in Methow Valley, Washington, about a five-hour drive from Seattle.

It just so happened that the East Coast was slammed by a nor'easter of epic proportions at the exact same time that Arun was trying to get home to Seattle. The blizzard had grounded air traffic, impacting cities from Philadelphia to Providence.

As I cried to Arun that I didn't want to miss our vacation and that our lodge accommodations were nonrefundable, I had no idea that he intended to bring an engagement ring out of hiding in the Methow Valley.

There was nothing else for Arun to do but wait. He spent days at the airport, hoping to secure a standby seat. Flights kept getting canceled. Finally, in the 11th hour, the gate agent called his name, and he practically sprinted to board that plane.

All was not lost!

Memoirs of a Surgeon's Wife, by Megan Sharma

We made it to the pristine snowscape of the Methow Valley, where the skies were clear, and the hot tub was extra hot. Never mind that you had to wear snow boots and a robe and sprint to the jacuzzi in sub-zero temperatures. That was all part of the fun.

Exactly two years after our first date, December 30, we set out on a snowshoe adventure. We couldn't find the right trail and got yelled at profusely for accidentally venturing onto a cross country skiing trail. Well, excuuuse us.

Eventually, we found ourselves on a lovely valley floor trail circling the lodge property. The scenery was breathtaking-literally. It kind of hurt to breathe, because of the cold. But it was amazing.

When it became clear that we had almost completed the trail loop (time running out), Arun suddenly stopped in the path front of me. He started saying all kinds of nice things, and I knew immediately that he was about to propose.

He got down on one knee. In the snow. The frigid snow. He said, "And that's why I am about to ask you to marry me." I immediately screamed, "YES!!!" And then he asked, "Will you marry me?" and I said "YES!!!" for a second time.

Even now, we still joke about his confusing phrasing, and why he felt the need to first notify me that he was *going to* propose, and then actually propose in the next breath.

It was just perfect. And the best part was that we were miles and miles from a cell phone signal, so we could just bask in the glory of our new engagement without the obligation to immediately call our entire family and set of friends. We did, however, call our parents via calling card, who were all "on high alert," and absolutely thrilled for us.

Where there's a will, there's a way. And a word of advice to men planning to propose while snowshoeing: practice kneeling in the snow. I hear it's not that easy to pull off.

Memoirs of a Surgeon's Wife, by Megan Sharma

DR. AND MRS.

The night before our wedding, as I tried my hardest to get some shuteye, I was thwarted again and again by the incessant lyrics of "Desi Girl" running through my head. Unless you are Indian, you probably don't know the song I'm referring to. If you are Indian, you'll have the song stuck in your head for the next three days. (Sorry!) It was featured in a 2008 Bollywood movie, "Dostana," and is quite popular with Indian DJs.

Of course, most of the lyrics are in Hindi. My Hindi vocabulary is extremely limited, so I could only remember the English chorus about being the hottest girl in the world. It's a super catchy, bouncy, and repetitive song. Check it out on YouTube and you'll see what I mean.

When I woke up on my wedding morning after only three hours of precious sleep, my Maid of Honor and best friend, Melinda, who had stayed with me on my last night as an unmarried woman, asked how I had slept. Not well, Melinda! Not well.

But it was worth it. You see, we had partied hard the night before. No, it wasn't for my bachelorette party. And by "partied hard" I mean that we had the time of our lives, and we were not drunk.

It was our Mehndi party. A Mehndi/Sangeet is a traditional Indian pre-wedding event that feels very much like an energetic wedding reception, with a few cool twists. "Mehndi" refers to henna, which is provided for all the women at the party. Since my mehndi took several hours to apply to my hands and feet (it was stunning!), I had already done mine earlier in the week.

Memoirs of a Surgeon's Wife, by Megan Sharma

Everyone wears traditional Indian clothing: saris, suits (tunic and leggings) and lehengas (top and skirt) for the ladies, and kurta pajamas (not actually pajamas—a dressy men's outfit) for the men. My family donned Indian clothes for the occasion, as well.

The Mehndi includes gifts of bangles (bracelets) and bindis (small forehead jewel stickers) for the women. There is food, enough food to feed a small town. We chose beach themed buffet stations. But the main event is the dancing.

I had never attended a Mehndi before my own, so I didn't know what to expect. After dinner is served, a whole program of family dance performances unfolds. It begins with the oldest generation and proceeds from there to the youngest. Arun's amazing grandmother, our mummiji, loves to dance. She kicked off the performances in style. She was 87 at the time, mind you.

Then were the dances from Arun's parents, aunts and uncles, and cousins. All themed and enthusiastically performed. Some people look a bit silly when they dance, but they do so with such abandon that you cannot help but smile and share in their joy.

By the end of the performances, everyone was ready to get up and move. We had asked our Indian DJ to give a brief dance lesson for all our friends and family, to help everyone get into the party spirit. So, we all learned a dance to "Jai Ho" with DJ Prashant.

And then Arun and I surprised everyone with our own dance performance: choreographed together in our living room. Arun had been practicing obsessively, so it went off without a hitch. Well, until the DJ kept playing the song after our dance ended. We just kept dancing. And at that point everyone joined us.

To say that we all had a blast would be a huge understatement. We danced our little hearts out. All of us—young and old, Indian and American. It was the ultimate start to our wedding weekend.

Now we were going to get married! OMG!

Despite my lack of sleep, I was filled with excitement and could not wait to finally say "I do." Throughout the course of the wedding day, which was an unusually sunny May day in Seattle, my family and bridesmaids made several

Memoirs of a Surgeon's Wife, by Megan Sharma

comments about being surprised or impressed with how calm I was. I am a super detail-oriented, type A person who tends to worry over things—hence, their shock.

I was at peace. We had been planning this freakin' wedding with not one, but two wedding planners for nearly a year and a half, and it was time to get the show on the road. Once our relatives began arriving from the U.K., India, and across the United States and our wedding events kicked off with bridesmaid day, our rehearsal dinner and Arun's bachelor party, we sort of both took a deep breath, looked at one another and said, "Ok, let's go. Time to enjoy our wedding." And we did.

All our planning for multiple events and somehow combining two very different cultural backgrounds paid off. We heard about some snafus after the fact, like a bridesmaid dress that didn't fit and a trip to the hospital for a sick little girl, but we thoroughly enjoyed all the moments of our wedding weekend.

Anyway, back to the wedding morning.

So, yes, I was a mother-f-ing-Zen-master on my wedding day. The only time I had to take a moment to remember to inhale and exhale was right before my first look with Arun. I don't know why I was nervous—it certainly wasn't about getting married. Arun is the love of my life, no question about it. It was more like, "I hope my soon-to-be-husband thinks I look really hot in my wedding dress!" As soon as I saw him, I was again chill as a cucumber.

And so, the day unfolded. Photos on the waterfront with an unexpected tugboat festival (what???) and sunburns all around for the unprepared bridal party dressed in strapless gowns (myself included). Riding in a vintage white Rolls Royce with my love to the photoshoot location and to the wedding venue, waving at passersby like Princess Diana. Arriving at the wedding venue and casually watching from the upper level, unseen, as our guests streamed in. Skylights giving the ceremony a truly ethereal feel. Ribbons everywhere in royal purple, tiffany blue, fuchsia and white. Me getting so anxious right before the ceremony (stage fright, really), that I had to run in place to the tune of "Maniac" and act like a total weirdo just to keep my makeup intact. Walking down the aisle with my dad, who somehow was completely composed and made sure that I wasn't walking too fast. The strange sensation of having over 100 people staring at me in unison. Representing both our heritages with a combined Christian and Hindu ceremony—with Arun's dad performing the Hindu ceremony. Both of our parents and my brother actively participating in the Hindu ceremony to give their blessings. Trying to make sure my

Memoirs of a Surgeon's Wife, by Megan Sharma

wedding gown (a billowy strapless ball gown in a shimmery shade of blush) didn't go up in flames from the Havan fire as I walked the seven circles with Arun, representing our seven vows of love to one another. Focusing on Arun and watching his face—his eyes full of love and his lip quivering ever so slightly with emotion during our personally chosen wedding vows. Our first kiss as Dr. and Mrs. and our triumphant entrance into married life. We did it!

After the ceremony, we changed into our traditional Indian wedding outfits. Both were exceptionally bling-tastic, hand sewn with thousands of beads and jewels and of the finest silk in India. Arun looked like a prince. I guess I looked snazzy myself in my fuchsia lehenga with gold stitching. The skirt alone weighed 25 pounds. We danced to "Somebody like You" by Keith Urban for our first dance, our mummiji (Arun's grandmother) cutting in to bless us. We feasted on incredible Indian and American dishes like mutter paneer with basmati rice and truffle cream mac n cheese. And then there were the speeches. We were blown away by all of them. The cleverest of all was Arun's younger brother and Best Man, Amar, who delivered this line so well that we thought Jimmy Fallon would have been jealous: (talking about how great Arun is) "He's also so hard working, so smart, so…hmmm…sorry, Arun Bhaiya (brother), I can't read your handwriting." Pause for effect.

We danced, and we danced some more. We hugged our friends and family and tried to drink in every fleeting moment. When it was finally time to head off into the moonlight for our wedding night, we rushed through a tunnel of brightly colored streamers waved by our loved ones to yet another model of vintage white Rolls Royce. Before heading back to our hotel, we took a scenic drive on Alki Beach and enjoyed our first moments alone together in about 12 hours. We re-lived the highlights reel in our hotel room and ate Vietnamese noodle salad at 2 am.

I will also mention that we nearly didn't make it to our honeymoon the next morning, and not because of a failed alarm.

We were set to leave for the Big Island of Hawaii. We had packed everything with us at the local hotel but wanted to return our wedding garments to our condo, less than two miles away. It was supposed to be a quick drop off and head to the airport type of scenario.

Instead, we found all the streets around our condo closed off for some sort of running race. And I mean ALL the streets. We went from block to block searching for a possible entrance but finding none within three blocks of our condo. These are three city blocks—large ones, interlaced with one-way streets.

Memoirs of a Surgeon's Wife, by Megan Sharma

We finally thought we found a street to break through when a police car suddenly started backing toward us and nearly hit us. The guy was a total a-hole as we tried to explain our predicament. Literally no help at all.

Running out of time, we parked three or four blocks from our condo, grabbed our extremely heavy and bulky collection of wedding outfits—wedding dress, Mehndi lehenga and wedding lehenga for me, and three outfits for Arun—and sprinted down the street with our heavy burdens. We even had to run through the race at one point, waiting for the crowd to part.

Fearing we would miss our flight, we parked in the most expensive section of the parking garage just adjacent to the terminal. Oy.

But we made it! And Hawaii was everything we dreamed it would be. Sea turtles, helicopter ride over a volcano, open air restaurants serving fresh-plucked Ono, and more.

That's the story of how we became Dr. and Mrs. Sharma.

Memoirs of a Surgeon's Wife, by Megan Sharma

MY WONDERFUL INDIAN FAMILY

This may come as a shock: I was not born Indian. My maiden name is Marsh. As in a swampy bog, or something of that nature.

Ancestry.com has revealed that I am 28% Irish/Scottish/Welsh, 25% Scandinavian, 24% British, 13% from the Iberian Peninsula (Spain and Portugal), and 10% from other regions. So, I guess the whole swampy bog thing makes sense.

Until I met my husband, I had very little exposure to Indian culture. I think I'd eaten Indian food once. So...I was not prepared for the awesomeness that would ensue.

The Sharma family is, hands down, the best Indian family in these United States, and that is an irrefutable fact. I seriously love my big, boisterous Indian family.

Here is my top 10 countdown for why Indian families (and mine, in particular) rock:

10. Gifts. Indians are very generous and love to give gifts for many occasions, such as when visiting someone's home, when you haven't seen a friend or family member for some time, to commemorate a holiday, to celebrate a new job or promotion, and of course, for weddings and babies. My favorite part is that for gifts of money, an extra $1 is always thrown in for good luck. It just seems like a good idea, right?

Memoirs of a Surgeon's Wife, by Megan Sharma

9. Festivals and holidays. Indians have the best holidays! There are more than 30 Hindu holidays in each year (Wikipedia, 2016). Some of my favorites are Holi, the festival of colors, when Indians chase one another through the streets and get covered in bright powdered colors of the rainbow. Another lovely holiday is Karva Chauth, when married women fast from sunrise to moonrise and pray for the longevity of their husbands, and then enjoy a special meal together. There is also Rakhi, which celebrates brotherly and sisterly love and gives siblings a chance to bless one another for the coming year. The best of all is Diwali, perhaps the most famous of Indian holidays: the festival of lights. It's like Christmas and Independence Day all rolled into one. Arun and I were lucky enough to spend Diwali in Agra in 2012 with our family. There were prayers, an elaborate and delicious home cooked meal, houses decorated everywhere with lights and vibrant yellow and orange marigold flowers, and a sizable arsenal of fireworks, which still didn't scare away the monkeys who laid claim to the terrace. Fun times!

8. Sweets. Oh, boy, do I have a sweet tooth. The good and the bad of it is that eating Mithai (sweets) is intrinsic to Indian culture. It seems to be in the DNA. Any celebratory occasion includes a variety of sweets, often containing milk, sugar, cardamom, cashews and pistachios. A few of my top Mithai picks are Gulab Jamun, which is like a donut soaked in sugary rosewater. My father-in-law, Prabhakar, also makes a delightful Kheer (Indian rice pudding). But you pretty much can't go wrong with any of them. And it's rude to refuse, so...I eat it all. The sacrifices I make.

7. An international family. The Sharma family lives all around the world, from the U.S. to England and India. It's always a blast when we get together and try to decipher one another's slang.

6. Fashion. Indian clothes are remarkable, especially for special occasions. Luminous colors and fabrics, hand bead and stone work, hand stitched embroidery—every piece is unique. I always look forward to the opportunity to shop for and wear Indian garments. My mother-in-law, Jyoti, also does a fabulous job of choosing pieces for me when she visits India. Thanks, Jyoti! You're the best!

5. Incredible India. Being part of an Indian family means that you may have the opportunity to visit India. If you do, take it! India truly is an incredible place. It's a feast for the senses. Everywhere you look, life is just bursting at the seams. There is so much color and character and so many animals roaming around freely (cows, dogs, monkeys, camels, water buffalo, you name it!). It doesn't compare to anywhere else in the world.

Memoirs of a Surgeon's Wife, by Megan Sharma

4. Food. You have not lived until you've eaten Jyoti's chicken biryani (Indian fried rice), bhindi (okra), chole bhature—Arun's favorite—(chickpea curry with fried bread), daal (cooked lentils), and dosa (crunchy South Indian pancakes filled with potatoes or onions). Uh oh. I'm having a serious food craving!

3. Weddings. Indian weddings are the bomb. Indians sure know how to party and love to dance, no matter their age. Arun's grandmother, Mummiji, who is now in her 90s, is always on the dance floor at weddings. There are also plenty of events to keep the celebration going for several days at a time. At a minimum, there is the Sangeet/Mehndi, which is basically like a big wedding reception, but with a bonus of family choreographed dance performances and henna (mehndi) for the women. And then, of course, there is an elaborate wedding ceremony and a huge wedding reception. Weddings are a family reunion for us, and we eagerly look forward to them!

2. Strong tradition and values. India and Hinduism boast thousands of years of history and rich culture. There is always something more to learn, and lessons that can be applied to our modern lives. What I appreciate about the Sharma family is their dedication to supporting one another and to spending time together. Nothing is more important than family.

1. Your family is my family. For Indians, the concept of family is a fluid one. It can include family friends, neighbors, extended family and in-laws. Any member of your extended family is warmly welcomed. Anyone could be your "uncle" or "auntie." And if you don't know or remember their name when you see them, you're just fine calling them that. It's a tight knit community that welcomes even those who hail from swampy bogs (Marshes).

Memoirs of a Surgeon's Wife, by Megan Sharma

MYTH BUSTERS: MEDICINE AND HOLY MATRIMONY

Doctors and their families live the glamourous life, yes? Black tie charity galas. Golfing at Pebble Beach. Hob knobbing with celebrities and politicians. Wheels up to exotic locations on our private jet. Shopping sprees at Chanel and Prada. Regular features in the gossip columns. Special treatment like reservations at the hottest Manhattan restaurants. Full staff of live-in nannies, landscapers, man-scapers, and personal assistants. Miniature poodles toted in Louis Vuitton purses. A butler named Jeeves who lives in our pantry, sitting patiently cross-legged and white gloved, just waiting for the opportunity to offer us chocolate almond bark and Darjeeling tea. A collection of sports cars. A bevy of spectacular summer homes from the Hamptons to Honolulu, and, of course—a supersize yacht or two.

The reality is far less enchanting and certainly not worthy of the Kennedys.

We are regular people. We watch reality TV. We take our daughter to swim lessons at the YMCA. We shop at Target—way too much. We rarely spend more than $10 on a bottle of wine. We love to use our Papa Bucks at Papa Murphy's Take N Bake pizza. We giggle, we cry, we sometimes burp out loud. We go to play dates. We love a good country music concert. We send Christmas cards (late!) bearing photos of our daughter. We wear our tennis shoes until they are absolutely destroyed. Until recently, we owned an older Honda Accord without a built-in navigation system or a back-up camera. We procrastinate on cleaning our garage. We fear the day our daughter will set off for college and leave us behind.

If we lived on the Upper East Side or in LA proper, it might be a completely different picture because lifestyle and appearances are much more "important" in places like that. But that's just not who we are, and not where we came from.

Arun and I both come from humble beginnings.

Arun was born in Bathinda, India and moved to the United States at the tender age of five. Adorably, he thought that he and his parents could simply take a taxi to America. It wasn't as easy as that, unfortunately. But he did quite enjoy the soda he shared with his parents—his first ever—while waiting at the U.S. Embassy. He arrived in the U.S. on Halloween day, and was terrified upon seeing all the people in costume and not understanding what in the world was going on.

Life in India was not easy. His parents did not own a car or a TV. They did own a scooter and would often ride on it together as a family of three through chaotic Indian traffic riddled with livestock, many other families and young couples on scooters, buses carrying passengers hanging out windows and riding on the rooftop, and plenty of foot traffic.

The Sharma family home, like most others, did not consistently have hot water. Electricity was spotty, at best. Bathing was from a bucket.

Because refrigeration wasn't exactly reliable, Arun's grandmother walked every day to get fresh milk for him. Cooking was done for every meal and with considerable effort. There was no microwave.

The entire family, all three generations, lived together in a small home. It didn't seem to be too tiny at the time, but years later Arun and his father returned to the home in India and couldn't imagine how they'd all lived there happily, shoulder to shoulder.

Arun's parents wanted more than anything to raise Arun and his future brother in America, the land of opportunity. When they finally arrived in New Jersey in 1987, they might as well have landed on Mars. Everything was completely different from the life they knew in India: language, people, culture, customs, cost of living, and the career world. And they weren't surrounded by all the loved ones who made up their strong support system back home.

Memoirs of a Surgeon's Wife, by Megan Sharma

Although both Jyoti (Arun's mom) and Prabhakar (Arun's dad) were highly educated and already on a successful career path, translating that success in America was not as straightforward as they might have hoped. It took time and determined effort.

As more family members began to emigrate to America, the Sharmas opened their home. They lived in a small apartment together and never complained about needing privacy or more space. In fact, for most of his childhood years, Arun shared a bedroom with his grandmother.

Today, the American dream has become a reality for the Sharma family. Prabhakar and Jyoti have built solid and accomplished careers and have provided generously for their two sons, allowing both to pursue their unique dreams.

While I was born in America and had a very different upbringing from Arun, we share many commonalities at the core of our childhood experience.

I am also the oldest child in our family, born in the heart of Silicon Valley, California in the early 1980s. My parents married young after a whirlwind courtship and my mom gave birth to me when she was only 23. We were never rich. Growing up, my parents rented housing in the Bay Area until they could purchase their first home in Sacramento with an astronomical mortgage interest rate of over nine percent.

It didn't take much to content my two brothers and me. We loved playing on our backyard swing set, making up circus-like routines and planning to sell admission tickets for our show to friends and family. There wasn't a Sacramento summer day that went by without us splashing around our above ground "doughboy" pool for hours on end. Sometimes we even shared the pool with our Springer Spaniel, Oreo.

Our entertainment mainly consisted of swimming, riding bikes, and playing games with our neighborhood and church friends. We also played poker and gin rummy with our Grandma Pearson, who taught us everything we know about cards. We were thrilled when we received a Nintendo game system and could play Super Mario Brothers, with one of us dancing in a circle or hanging upside down from our parents' bed to muster enough good luck to complete the level.

Memoirs of a Surgeon's Wife, by Megan Sharma

We never took extravagant vacations and we definitely never stayed in hotels—not even the Holiday Inn. What we did was essentially free if you discount the cost of gas and food: we went camping. We had a camper on the back of our pickup truck and enjoyed the great outdoors all over Northern California, from the redwoods to the Pacific. I think that's part of the reason why I have such a deep love and appreciation of nature.

Even as I reached teenage years, we never went to Disneyland or other typical American vacations (sorry, mom! I had to mention it!). We did visit local amusement parks and water parks frequently. And we did drive from Seattle to San Jose, a 14 to 15-hour trip, about once a year. Anyone who has made this voyage in the back of a minivan with two brothers, a set of parents and at least one pungent Golden Retriever will attest that it is the opposite of relaxing.

When I was 16, I was commanded to go out and get a job, despite my lack of experience with anything other than babysitting. I began working at Old Navy on evenings and weekends when I wasn't attending school (including AP classes), studying, going to church, volunteering and cheerleading.

You see, even though Arun and I grew up thousands of miles from one another, we shared many values that we had learned growing up: the values of hard work, determination, education, making something out of nothing, and appreciating what is important in life: family.

We both had happy and productive childhoods, and for that we will be forever grateful to our loving parents and grandparents, who took the time to help build our character, a task much easier said than done.

We didn't have trust funds. We didn't have silver platters. Our children won't get that kind of legacy, and that is a promise.

I guess you could say that this myth of a perfect, groomed doctor's life has been busted.

Memoirs of a Surgeon's Wife, by Megan Sharma

PART 3: LIFE IN THE TRENCHES: RESIDENCY

❖ ❖ ❖ ❖ ❖

Memoirs of a Surgeon's Wife, by Megan Sharma

A HAIKU FOR EVERY SEASON

The Japanese tradition of haiku focuses on nature, simplicity and expression of powerful emotions. Seasons often come into play and help illustrate the mood of the poet.

There is a season for every step in the journey of a physician, as well.

The dream of becoming a doctor
Save the world, I will
Cancer is no match for me
Oops, here comes the bill

Medical school
Here I learn the ropes
Study, study, study, CRASH
Blood stains on my shoes

Residency
I'm a doctor, yo
Show me some respect, I beg
How old am I, now?

Finishing residency
There's the finish line
Gave it all my heart and soul
Pager by my side

Fellowship
One more year ahead
Time to take a flying leap

Memoirs of a Surgeon's Wife, by Megan Sharma

Hello, baby girl

First real job
Can it truly be?
I got a real job, you guys!
Best is yet to come

Memoirs of a Surgeon's Wife, by Megan Sharma

THE ROAD TO M.D.

I was poking around our shared files while working on this book when I happened upon a folder called "Med School Applications" with a photo of a young, glossy haired, earnest looking version of my hubby. Hand, meet cookie jar.

Now, he has told me before why he wanted to become a doctor. Essentially, he sought to cure cancer and save the world. Totally doable. Although, as a child, he wanted to become the President of the United States *and* an astronaut. Space President, if you will. Presiding over the United States and the moon. He was devastated to learn that the POTUS must be a natural-born U.S. citizen. I guess medicine was the back-up career.

I did feel slightly guilty snooping around Arun's personal documents. But I must say that right away I was super impressed with how polished and well-written his essays were. I'm not surprised—he is very intelligent and has always been a good writer (he was the Editor-in-Chief of the Hopkins Undergraduate Research Journal (HURJ), as he likes to remind me).

Just to give you an idea of the type of person he is and why his patients are fortunate to have him, I'll quote from a few of those essays.

Arun described his experience volunteering with ChildLife in glowing terms: "Most of the children I see are recovering from various surgical operations. By playing games, reading books, and simply talking with them, I can help them feel better mentally and emotionally. Although I have no discrete evidence to support this statement, I would also venture to say that by simply making them happier, I am sure that I have also helped with their physical recoveries."

Memoirs of a Surgeon's Wife, by Megan Sharma

He goes on to say: "For me, the allure of a medical career comes from knowing that I will be able to directly improve the physical health of patients in addition to their mental and emotional health, as I am able to now. Whether teaching a child how to multiply, reading books with a recovering child, or operating on a patient, the joy of knowing that I have made someone's life better is something that would keep me motivated regardless of the obstacles presented to me."

That is just so sweet. I love this guy.

As will be shocking to no one, Arun got into his top choice medical school with a full scholarship. BOOM.

Memoirs of a Surgeon's Wife, by Megan Sharma

AN INTRODUCTION TO SURGICAL RESIDENCY

First things first: The New England Journal of Medicine describes surgery as "a profession defined by its authority to cure by means of bodily invasion." (Atul Gawande, 2012) I think we can all agree that opening a living person's body is not something to be undertaken casually!

For that reason and many others, surgeons are highly trained and educated.

Four years of undergraduate study in subjects such as biology, physics or chemistry, successful completion of the Medical College Admission Test (MCAT) to apply to medical school, acceptance to medical school, four to five years of deeper study and hands-on experience with patients in medical school, and at that point the coveted Doctor of Medicine (M.D.) title is earned. Then, there is a required residency program.

This is an incredibly competitive field in the U.S. Of the 53,042 individuals who applied to U.S. medical schools for 2016-2017, less than 40 percent were accepted. On average, each person submitted applications to 16 schools (AAMC, 2016).

Let's talk about residency, the next step after medical school. The concept of a formal medical residency was pioneered at The Johns Hopkins University in the late 1800s and early 1900s by William Osler (Johns Hopkins Medicine, 2014). The term residency stems from the reality that many physicians spent most of their time "in house," or physically in the hospital, often for days at a time. The hospital became their home away from home.

Memoirs of a Surgeon's Wife, by Megan Sharma

The length of surgical residency varies from specialty to specialty, typically from three to eight years. For Otolaryngology (also known as Ear Nose and Throat—ENT) surgeons like my husband, residency is a five-year endeavor, sometimes six. Plus, an additional year or two of research during residency that technically doesn't "count" as an official post-graduate year.

That's right, six years in the prime of life (mid-twenties to early thirties), working harder than any medical student ever imagined possible.

Just when you think you've crossed the finish line, you see it still looming in the distance. For those surgeons who want to pursue an academic career, perhaps in a university hospital setting, rather than in private practice, a post-residency fellowship is essential. Fellowships are generally one to two years in length, depending on the amount of research involved.

All in all, when my husband finally finished his surgical ENT residency and one-year fellowship in 2015, he had 16 years of post-high school education under his belt, in addition to a few unwelcome gray hairs, as a nifty bonus.

Sixteen years: that's the equivalent of a driving teenager, and the level of education achieved by only 1.32 percent of the U.S. population over 18 years of age (United States Census Bureau, 2012).

Commitment? I'll say! Chutzpah? Hell yes!

Memoirs of a Surgeon's Wife, by Megan Sharma

NO SCRUBS

TLC (the incomparable "CrazySexyCool" girl group) refused to lower themselves to the level of a guy who can't pay his bills but somehow still thinks that he can hit on women. Great relationship advice is timeless, am-I-right?

I don't want no scrubs, either. But I am talking about medical issue wardrobe, not broke dudes.

When we first started dating, I thought it was fun to wear Arun's scrub bottoms as pajama pants, sometimes in public. Oh, look at me! I'm dating a doctor! Megan, *you adorable idiot*. I grew disillusioned when our condo became overrun with wrinkled, dirty masses of cheap cotton in various shades of steel blue and jade green.

My initial strategy was to wash and fold them myself. This was annoying, as it clogged our washer and dryer and overall seemed like an exercise in futility. And then, my moment of Zen: I realized that there is a service at each hospital that washes scrubs for FREE! Enough of this.

I then issued an official directive to Arun to start returning the scrubs to work for cleaning on a regular basis. What happened instead: piles of dirty scrubs in our condo, "ready" to go out the door. Ready and waiting. And waiting. And W-A-I-T-I-N-G...

The offending scrubs were moved to Trader Joe's bags at the back of our parking garage space. Until the building got wise and posted a notice in the elevator to keep parking spaces clear. From there, the overstuffed Trader Joe's bags traveled the short distance to the trunk of Arun's car. Well, a car trunk only has so much room.

Memoirs of a Surgeon's Wife, by Megan Sharma

The scrubs eventually reached their final resting place: either the hospital from whence they came, or a dumpster. (Sorry! not sorry! you would do the same.)

Arun's fellowship program in Pittsburgh had the right idea: to get new scrubs, you had to return the old ones via a vending machine, and you were only allowed three at a time. This institution clearly understood human nature. Our Pittsburgh apartment was always dirty-scrub-pile-free!

My takeaway lesson? Scrubs can multiply faster than you can say drawstring, so new boyfriends and girlfriends of medical professionals, beware!

Memoirs of a Surgeon's Wife, by Megan Sharma

THE IRONIES OF BEING A SURGICAL RESIDENT

Alanis Morissette's iconic 1995 hit song, "Ironic," is proof positive that life is often darkly humorous and patently unfair. I will forever love that song and sing the chorus at the top of my lungs, my voice cracking on the high notes (just like every other girl of my generation).

The ironies of life as a surgical resident are plenty. "Days off" are spent preparing for cases, writing or dictating patient notes, fielding phone calls from junior residents or attendings, working on statistics and research, and, if there's time left over, making sure there is at least one clean pair of underwear in your dresser drawer.

Doctors encourage their patients to live healthy lifestyles, complete with balanced eating, exercise, and regular check-ups with their primary care provider. Yet, they can't find the time to do these things for themselves. Who has time for a doctor appointment when they work 80 hours (+) a week?

Everyone seems to think that doctors are filthy rich. In fact, residents (who are officially doctors) are squeaky poor, especially when they reside in a city with high cost of living, like Seattle.

Alanis, perhaps you should consider a reprise on "Ironic" to include some of these little gems. Have your people call my people.

Memoirs of a Surgeon's Wife, by Megan Sharma

THE REALITY OF BEING "ON CALL"

Rather than explaining in detail the rather obvious reality of what it means to be "on call," I would like to offer some advice for residents on what NOT to do while on call:

1. Staff a telethon for a beloved charity
2. Enter a hot dog eating contest, and win
3. Catch up with a verbose grandmother
4. Take a long, luxurious bubble bath
5. Cook your way through Julia Child's "Mastering the Art of French Cooking"
6. Hike in terrain outside of cell phone range
7. Retrieve a distant relative with dubious accommodation plans from the airport
8. Attempt to get a killer deal at the local used car dealership
9. Go on a city-wide pub crawl
10. Audition for a TV endorsement deal for a hot new dietary supplement

Memoirs of a Surgeon's Wife, by Megan Sharma

UNWRITTEN RULES OF THE OR

To surgeons, the operating room (OR) is the like the biblical Holy of Holies: it's a sacred place. Like any hallowed ground, it has a bevy of rules, many of them unspoken. I won't get too much into technicalities here, but this will give you a flavor of life in the OR.

Here is an OR primer for the uninitiated:

1. Cover it up: be sure your head and facial hair, in addition to your entire body, are completely covered with proper attire. This includes facial mask, scrub cap for your head, a 'bunny suit' to go over your scrubs, and shoe covers.

2. NO TOUCHING: seriously, don't touch anything. Keep your hands to yourself. The goal of the operating room is to maintain sterility to reduce the possibility of infection.

3. Keep your distance: stand several feet away from the sterile (surgical) field. Unless you are performing or assisting with the surgery, of course.

4. Zip the lip: don't speak unless spoken to in the OR. People's lives are at stake and unnecessary conversation can be a dangerous distraction. Yet, music isn't necessarily out of the question. My hubby prefers to listen to the Hip Hop BBQ Pandora station while operating, but everyone has their preferences. He now has a reputation for being quite "gangsta." Go figure.

5. Know why you're there: if you are a medical student or a resident (or any member of the surgical team, for that matter), you should know who the patient is and why we are performing surgery on them. This sounds so Captain Obvious that you would think it's not even worth mentioning, but it's easy to overlook in the mad rush of surgical life.

Ready to slice and dice? Me, neither.

Memoirs of a Surgeon's Wife, by Megan Sharma

MISSION: STRESS RELIEF

In Arun's line of work, as you can imagine, there is a fair amount of stress. We're talking about life and death, here.

And sometimes it can get a tad heavy, even for me.

"Sorry to be a Debbie Downer," Arun will say, after he's told me the most heart-wrenching story of all time. Too late, husband! Too late! I am down. And you are Debbie.

One of our favorite stress relief techniques is a little unorthodox.

We simply tune our Pandora station to "Mauja Hi Mauja" or bhangra radio, crank it up, and dance around the living room like crazy fools. Sometimes we feel the need to don some stunna shades. It helps with the attitude adjustment.

Change the lightbulb, pat the dog. Change the lightbulb, pat the dog. That's how Bollywood style dance was initially explained to me. Anyone can do the basics.

You simply cannot feel bummed out when you are dancing to Indian music! Our secret Bollywood dance parties are an awesome stress reliever.

Forget the spin bike. Jai ho!

Memoirs of a Surgeon's Wife, by Megan Sharma

THE 80-HOUR WORKWEEK: DAMNED IF YOU DO, DAMNED IF YOU DON'T

The 40-hour workweek, aka "the grind," is the American standard. It's been that way by law since 1940, when Congress amended the Fair Labor Standards Act (the Act was initially passed in 1938 with a workweek of 44 hours) (Lebowitz, 2015).

Yet, we all know that salaried professionals regularly work more than 40 hours per week. The expectation is to get the job done, period.

What you may not know is that today there are no legal limits to the number of hours a medical resident can work. I repeat, NO LEGAL LIMITS. There are limits, but they are not enforceable by law.

However, in 2003, things got a bit brighter for medical residents in the United States. The Accreditation Council for Graduate Medical Education (ACGME), the powerful private organization responsible for accrediting medical residency and fellowship programs nationwide, instituted duty hour requirements.

Duty hours are "all clinical and academic activities related to a program; that is: patient care (both inpatient and outpatient); administrative duties relative to patient care; the provision for transfer of patient care; time spent in-house during call activities; and scheduled activities, such as conferences. Duty hours do not include reading and preparation time spent away from the duty site." (ACGME, 2016)

The key requirement stipulates that residents are not to exceed 80 hours per week of duty hours, averaged over four weeks (ACGME, 2016).

It's important to note that those 80 hours do *not* include activities performed away from the hospital (often at home), such as studying anatomy or case reports, preparing for surgery, writing patient notes, preparing updates for attending physicians, reviewing lab work and CT scans, responding to emails and text messages, studying for board examinations, and a million other things that add up to countless additional hours of ghost labor.

Why did the ACGME deem limited duty hours necessary? Officially, to "actualize the profession's social contract with society and compel Sponsoring Institutions to maintain an educational environment..." with safety and quality being paramount goals (ACGME, 2016).

Unofficially, just think about what working unlimited hours can do to a person.

Sleep deprivation. Stress. Anxiety. Depression. Substance abuse. Unhealthy eating patterns. Lack of exercise. Even suicide. The very least of these worries being the fact that work is life and life is work.

These are very real problems that can develop among incredibly smart and talented people. People who have dedicated their lives to helping others. People who have undertaken the enormous privilege and responsibility to become doctors.

The issue with the 80-hour workweek is this: it's unrealistic. Often, there is simply too much work and not enough manpower to complete it within 80 hours.

Let's take an example.

On a typical week as a resident, my husband would wake up at 4:00 or 5:00 a.m. to prepare for the day, check up on patients, etc. He would be at the hospital by 6:00 a.m. at the latest (usually sooner). So, let's just say that his work day "officially" began at 6:00 a.m.

Memoirs of a Surgeon's Wife, by Megan Sharma

There were many nights he would be stuck in a late surgery, staffing consults, putting in orders, making patient rounds, or simply catching up on patient care after surgery, and I didn't see him until 9:00 p.m. or later. However, for argument's sake, let's just say his average time 'clocking out' was 7:30 p.m. From 6:00 a.m. to 7:30 p.m. is a 13.5-hour day. Multiply that by five days, and you get 67.5 hours.

Now you should factor in call duties. Per ACGME standards, residents can take in-house call no more than once every three nights, averaged over four weeks (ACGME, 2016).

On a typical week, Arun was on call two days. Again, the amount of time spent on call only "counts" toward that 80 hours if it is spent at the duty site—if a resident goes in to see a patient or perform surgery.

The amount of time spent in the hospital varies greatly depending on the year of residency. Junior residents (interns, first and second year) are the first people to get paged and the most likely to spend almost all their time on call actively working at the hospital. More senior residents spend less time in the hospital because their junior colleagues are the first on the scene.

As a junior resident, Arun probably spent four to eight hours per call night at the hospital. Multiply eight hours times two nights, and that's 16 hours. Add 16 to the 67.5 standard workweek hours, and that's 83.5 hours.

ERRRRRRRRRRRRRRRRRRRRRRRRRRRRRRRRRRRRRRRRRRRRRRRR. The buzzer goes off. You're over your duty hours.

Where does that leave us?

Patient care cannot suffer. There is no resident fairy godmother to twirl her magic wand and make the work disappear. There is no one else to *do* the work. No one else is legally qualified or allowed to do the work.

This is where it gets sticky.

Institutions that violate the 80-hour workweek are penalized by the ACGME. They are penalized by taking away the most precious resource: people—residents for the program. If an institution violates the ACGME guidelines, they will be allowed less residents for the program the following year. ACGME also has the power to revoke residency program certification, which would be absolutely devastating to an institution.

This is more than a little backwards. There is obviously too heavy a workload, as evidenced by the number of hours required to get the job done. How will having less people to do the work solve the problem? Answer: it doesn't.

Because no residency or fellowship program wants to be penalized or discredited, an unspoken culture of fraud can develop. Residents are forced, often indirectly, to lie about their duty hours, so as not to hurt the program. But who wins in this situation?

A friend who is also a surgeon told me that when she was a resident, "No one cared if you didn't get the required time off. I and many junior residents were told to just lie about it, work from home, hide so that no one saw you—but to get the work done and to never mention that you only spent four to six hours away from the hospital."

Even worse, older surgeons who were not subject to the 80-hour workweek "in their day" are sometimes callous and view their younger trainees as weaker, or somehow less entitled to respect, simply because they are compelled to keep their average workweek to no more than DOUBLE the national average. Many of these senior attending physicians are more than a little vocal about their views, which puts residents in an awful position, and can even amount to harassment.

The perfect surgeon, after all, is one who never requires food, rest, or water. If you have time to eat you aren't working hard enough. Thus, many residents resort to scarfing half a PB&J sandwich in the bathroom, rather than face severe scrutiny and public shaming by senior residents for having the gall to want a meal once every 12 hours or so.

Essentially, the 80-hour workweek is a respectable idea. The intentions are admirable. But in practice, residents are damned if they do stay within 80 hours (only to be viewed as lazy or weak, with the potential to impact patient care), and damned if they don't (potentially harming the residency program in the future).

It's a catch 80. What is the solution?

Per the National Resident Matching Program (NRMP), the organization responsible for matching doctors to residency programs in the U.S., in 2016 there were 35,476 active applicants. Of these, 8,640 applicants—nearly 25 percent—were not matched to PGY-1 positions (the first year of residency) (NRMP, 2016). That's 8,640 dreams shattered, or potentially 8,640 missed opportunities.

The point is this: often, institutions could benefit from more residents in their programs, but cannot get them either due to budgetary constraints and/or being blocked by the ACGME. And there are many potentially qualified people out there who would absolutely love the job.

It's a complex issue. Obviously, you only want the very top-tier people in these positions, and the people who best fit the culture and environment of the residency program. Education is a top priority: this is where former medical students truly learn how to become doctors. There needs to be enough hands-on experience to go around.

Unfortunately, there is no silver bullet. But it's certainly worth further thought and consideration.

"Wherever the art of medicine is loved, there is also a love of humanity."—Hippocrates.

Memoirs of a Surgeon's Wife, by Megan Sharma

FACTS AND FIGURES: WHAT IT COSTS TO BECOME A SURGEON

Many people think that doctors, and surgeons especially, leak excess cash like water from a punctured waterbed. Yet, would-be doctors have to put up a ton of money just for the privilege of one day becoming one of the medical elite.

Not until much later in their careers will they make a reasonable salary—assuming they negotiate hard for what they deserve. In the process, it is possible and even highly likely for trainees to amass obscene amounts of debt, without careful planning and access to critical financial resources.

Many students simply have no idea what they're getting into.

Let's look at this step-by-step in the educational timeline.

- **College education at a four-year school. Data for 2016-2017:**
    - Published tuition and fees for *public* four-year schools average $9,650 per year (College Board, 2016)
    - Published tuition and fees for *private* nonprofit four-year schools average $33,480 per year (College Board, 2016)
    - I personally can vouch for the cost of attending a private, nonprofit school, which rang in at about $25,000 per year for tuition and fees when I attended Seattle Pacific University from 2001 to 2005. Got loans?

- So, the baseline price tag for a four-year college education is between $38,600 (public schools) and $133,920 (private nonprofit schools) as of 2016.
- And then there are those necessary expenses for room and board, books and supplies, transportation, and other cash vortexes that make up college life. The estimated 2016-17 budget for students attending either a public four-year school (in-state) or a private nonprofit four-year school, living on campus, is about $15,000 per year (College Board, 2016). A total added cost of $60,000 for four years.
- Let's assume that many pre-med students would opt for a private nonprofit school, simply to have an edge, and call the **total price tag for a four-year college education $193,920.**
  - **Note:** this is simply the price and does not factor in financial aid, scholarships, loans, and other methods of paying for college. It represents the "sticker price" to attend.

- **MCAT test prep courses and materials**
  - The Medical College Admission Test (MCAT) is the definitive test required for entry into U.S. medical schools.
  - The Association of American Medical Colleges (AAMC) sells the "Complete Official MCAT® Prep Bundle" for **$238** (AAMC, 2017).
  - MCAT prep courses: many people are not comfortable with self-study alone and opt to take an official MCAT prep course from providers such as Kaplan or The Princeton Review.
    - Kaplan offers 25 hours of MCAT private tutoring live online for about $4900 in the Seattle area (Kaplan, 2017).
    - Kaplan offers in-person classroom training for $2300-$2800 (Kaplan, 2017).
    - Kaplan offers self-paced online training for $2000-$2500 (Kaplan, 2017).
    - Let's assume the average person would choose an in-person classroom training series for **$2300.**
  - **Total cost: $2538**
- **MCAT exam registration fees**
  - Interestingly, MCAT exam registration fees are broken down in an Olympic medal-like system, with Gold, Silver, and Bronze Zone categories (AAMC, 2017).

- The Gold Zone favors those who plan ahead, allowing for registration up to one month or more prior to the exam, while the Bronze Zone "fly by seaters" can register one to two weeks prior to the exam, but pay a higher price, with no rescheduling or cancellation fees reimbursed.
- The base cost of initial registration is $310-$365
- Rescheduling the date and/or the test center costs $85-$145.
- So, for a test-taker who chooses the Silver Zone (right in the middle), the cost will be **$310** plus **$145** if they need to change the exam date or location.
- **Total cost: $455**

- **Medical school application fees**
  - There is a centralized system for medical school applications: the American Medical College Application Service® (AMCAS®).
  - For the 2017 application cycle, the AMCAS processing fee is **$160**, which includes one medical school designation. **Additional medical schools may be added at a cost of $38 each** (AAMC, 2017).
  - Per the AAMC, for 2016-2017 there were 830,016 medical school applications received from 53,042 applicants, an average of 16 applications per applicant (AAMC, 2016).
  - Assuming the 16-application standard, **total cost $730**

- **Medical school interviews: travel expenses**
  - "Most medical schools require an interview, though the process varies by school. Interviews can take place on or off campus. They can be conducted by one admissions committee member, by multiple members of the committee, or by off-campus interviewers, such as practicing physicians." (AAMC, 2017).
  - Let's use my husband as an example. Arun applied to 15 medical schools and interviewed in person, on campus at eight schools. He was a competitive candidate.
  - Arun was fortunate to live in Baltimore at the time and interviewed only at schools on the eastern seaboard. He drove to all interviews and did some couch surfing with family and friends, only staying one night in a hotel. His costs were minimal, mostly the cost of gas for the car and beer in exchange for a night's sleep.
  - However, many medical school applicants apply to schools all over the country. Naturally, these people pay a lot more to get to interviews: airfare, rental cars, and hotel stays.

Memoirs of a Surgeon's Wife, by Megan Sharma

- o   Because the range is so far and wide depending on a person's geographical starting point and how many schools they apply to, it's difficult to quantify the average cost of travel to medical school interviews.
- o   I will make some assumptions here. We'll continue with the understanding that the average person applies to 16 schools (AAMC, 2016). They likely will *not* get interviews at every one of these schools: let's say that a competitive candidate will get half: eight. This is simply an educated guess based on Arun's experience.
- o   Let's also assume that for these eight interviews, four will be local (within driving distance), and four will require a plane ticket.
- o   For the four interviews that require flying: average $400 round-trip per destination ($1600), plus three nights in a hotel at $150 per night in each location ($1800). Add $200 for rental car expenses per location ($800). Total is **$4200, and that's a conservative estimate**.
- o   For the four locally drivable locations, add **$400** in gas.
- o   **Total cost: $4600**

- **Medical school relocation expenses**
  - o   Unless you will attend medical school at the same college or university where you complete your undergraduate degree, you will be relocating to attend medical school after graduation.
  - o   Relocation expenses add up quickly:
    - Storage units (for in between time)
    - Packing supplies (think bubble wrap, packing tape and then some!)
    - Truck rentals (if doing it yourself)
    - Gas expenses (driving that truck)
    - Hotel expenses en route to your destination (depending on distance)
    - Hiring moving help for heavy lifting
    - Flying to far-away locations
    - Hiring movers to do it all
    - Shipping your car if you decide to fly
  - o   Again, with such a wide range of situations for the newly accepted medical school student moving to a new city, I will use my husband as an example. Arun moved from Baltimore, Maryland

Memoirs of a Surgeon's Wife, by Megan Sharma

to Pittsburgh, Pennsylvania to attend medical school at the University of Pittsburgh.

- Arun, being a little crazy (frugal), decided to drive the 250 miles between Baltimore and Pittsburgh not once, but twice, to move his things. That's 1,000 miles of driving, people! He did not rent a truck. He did not hire movers.
- He estimates $1000 total costs, including driving and new apartment purchases as follows: a desk, bed, chair, sofa, coffee table, bookshelf, and other basics. Add $600 for a new laptop. Arun's total expenses: **$1600**.
- You'll want to find a place to live before you move, so that will require a scouting visit. Let's assume $600 for airfare (for two people), $600 for hotel and $250 for a rental car, for a total of **$1450**.
- Assuming many med students would be in the same "starving student" mentality, we'll go with an average **total cost of $3,000** for relocation expenses. But for someone who chooses to fly, ship their car, and hire professional movers, the cost could be **$10,000**.
  - Average of these two options: **$6,500 total cost**.
- **Medical school education + loan interest over time**
  - Ah, medical school. That beacon of hope and desire for students the world over. It does not come at a bargain, my friends.
  - So, what does medical school cost? The median four-year cost of attendance for the class of 2017 is $240,351 for public schools and $314,202 for private schools. **Average cost: $277,277** (AAMC, 2017).
  - As of October 2016, 76 percent of all medical students graduate with educational debt. Of these, 82 percent graduate with $100,000 or more in debt (AAMC, 2016).
  - For the class of 2017, the median medical education debt is $180,000 (AAMC, 2016).
  - After graduation, it's nothing like a Kanye West video. The bling stops here: the median stipend for a first-year MD is $53,580 (AAMC, 2016).
  - Stop right there, Megan, you say. That's more money than I make! $50,000 is a good salary. And I totally hear you. The point I'm making here is that medical residents aren't making money in keeping with the number of hours they "officially" work (80+ per week) or the level of education they have achieved by

83

their first year of residency: a minimum of eight years after high school.
- ○ Also keep in mind this is a national stipend median—if you live in an expensive city like Seattle, your money will not go nearly as far. For example, you would need around $5,593 in Seattle to maintain the same standard of living you can have for $4,400 in Pittsburgh (assuming you rent in both cities). Compared to Pittsburgh, prices in Seattle are 66 percent higher for rent, 10 percent higher for restaurants, and 11 percent higher for groceries. (Numbeo, 2017).
- ○ And then there is the interest that comes along with the medical school debt. Again, the median debt is $180,000. Depending on interest rates and the terms of your loan, which vary greatly, you could be paying $92,000 to $227,000 in interest. **Average interest paid: $159,500.** (AAMC, 2016).
- ○ The average cost of medical school coupled with the average interest paid over time **grand total is: $436,777** (AAMC, 2016).

- **Residency program application fees**
  - ○ The next step in the educational journey is applying to a residency program during the fourth year of medical school (AKA—still broke).
  - ○ For 2016-2017, U.S. medical graduates applied to 55 residency programs, on average. International medical graduates applied to an average of 131.5 residency programs for the same academic year. (AAMC, 2017).
  - ○ Residency application fees are **$26 each** for 31 or more programs, plus a one-time fee of **$80** for USMLE transcript and **$80** for COMLEX-USA transcript, assessed once per season (AAMC, 2017).
  - ○ Let's limit ourselves to a discussion of U.S. medical graduates who have applied to 55 residency programs. At $26 a pop, that's **$1430**. Add the **$160** in transcript fees, and the **total is $1590**.
- **Residency program interviews: travel expenses**
  - ○ Medical students interview at about one-third of the residency programs to which they have applied (Benson, Stickle, & Raszka, 2015). With an average of 55 residency program applications per person, that works out to about 18 residency interviews.

Memoirs of a Surgeon's Wife, by Megan Sharma

- o Because the cost range for travel expenses to these interviews varies so much based on a person's geographical takeoff point, we need to make some assumptions to quantify the average cost.
- o Let's stick with the average of 18 interviews. Let's assume that five of the interviews will be local (within driving distance), and 13 will require a plane ticket.
- o For the 13 interviews that require flying: average $400 round-trip per destination ($5200), plus three nights in a hotel at $150 per night in each location ($5850), plus $200 for rental car in each location ($2600). **Total is $13,650, conservatively.**
- o For the five locally drivable locations, add **$500** in gas.
- o **Total cost: $14,150.**

- **Residency program relocation expenses**
  - o You got the job, woo hoo! Now you must pay to get yourself there. Unless you will complete your residency at the same college or university where you completed medical school, you will be relocating.
  - o Just like medical school relocation, the expenses are many: storage units, packing supplies, truck rentals, gas expenses, hotels, hired hands, plane tickets, and shipping your car.
  - o Again, it's essential to find a place to live before you move, so that will require a scouting visit. Let's assume $600 for airfare (for two people), $600 for hotel and $250 for a rental car, for a total of **$1450**.
  - o Because of the varying range of situations, I will again use Arun as an example. He moved from Pittsburgh, Pennsylvania to Seattle, Washington. This time there was no driving—he flew to Seattle and shipped his car. Since his furniture from med school wasn't much to speak of, he basically just moved himself, his clothing and other essentials—no furniture. Let's estimate the cost of new furniture (bedroom set, dining table and chairs, couch, chair, TV, TV stand, coffee table, 2 side tables, household accessories, large wardrobe since there was no closet, bookshelf, desk chair, etc.) at **$4000**—I roughly know what he paid for each item.
  - o Let's assume Arun paid **$300** for a one-way plane ticket. I happen to know that it costs about $1100 to ship a car from Seattle-Pittsburgh (since we did this years later), so the cost to ship his car from Pittsburgh to Seattle was **$1100**.

- ○ All in all, Arun's cost to move to Seattle was about **$6900**.
- ○ If a person chose to go all out and fly, ship their car and hire professional movers to do everything for them, it would cost $10,000.
- ○ Average of Arun's cheaper route and the full-service **total cost is $8450**.
- **State licensing fees during residency**
  - ○ Residents are practicing physicians. As such, they are required to pay state licensing fees for each year of residency.
  - ○ Want a leg up on the medical licensure requirements across the U.S.? The American Medical Association (AMA) offers an e-book, "State Medical Licensure Requirements and Statistics," revised annually and non-printable for $90, or $65 for AMA members (AMA, 2017).
  - ○ Arun's residency was six years, but he paid licensing for five years, since during his research year he did not practice.
  - ○ In Washington state, the Postgraduate Limited License fees specifically for residents are **$391** for the application and **$391** for annual license renewal (Washington State Department of Health, 2017). This means that Arun paid **$1955 total** for licensing during his residency. Of course, the cost varies by state.
- **Fellowship program application fees**
  - ○ For those who want to pursue an academic (university setting) surgical career, a fellowship is essential. Fellowships come after residency and are typically one to two years in length.
  - ○ The application fee for up to 10 programs is **$115**. Beyond that, additional applications are $11-26 each, plus a one-time fee of **$80** for USMLE transcript and **$80** for COMPLEX-USA transcript, assessed once per season (AAMC, 2017).
  - ○ **Total cost** for a person applying to 10 programs: **$275**.
- **Fellowship program interviews: travel expenses**
  - ○ Let's assume the average candidate would apply to 10 fellowship programs and receive interviews at five.
  - ○ Let's also assume that four out of five of those interviews require a plane ticket, while one is local (within driving distance).
  - ○ For the four interviews that require flying: average $400 round-trip per destination ($1600), plus three nights in a hotel at $150 per night in each location ($1800), plus $200 for rental car in each location ($800). **Total is $4200, conservatively**.
  - ○ For the one drivable location, add **$100** in gas.

Memoirs of a Surgeon's Wife, by Megan Sharma

- o Total: **$4300**.
- **Fellowship program relocation expenses**
  - o Time to hit the road again!
  - o I can use our experience as an example here. We moved from Seattle, Washington to Pittsburgh, Pennsylvania for Arun's fellowship year. We made a trip out to Pittsburgh before we moved to find a place to live. The rental car, gas, and hotel stay alone were about **$1000**. Add both of our round-trip plane tickets, another **$1000**.
  - o We were originally planning on driving the 2500 miles until a) we found out Arun only had about five days to move cross-country and start his new job, and b) I got pregnant and had unbearable nausea. We had no choice but to fly. We paid about $400 each for one-way tickets—total of **$800**.
  - o It cost **$1100** to ship our car out to Pittsburgh (we only had one car that we shared at the time).
  - o We did things the hard way and the cheap way because that was what we could afford. We packed everything ourselves and lived with my parents for two months after our condo sold and before Arun started his new job. Things added up very quickly, from packing materials and boxes to short term truck rental. We used two (exceptionally small!) U-Haul pods to get the entirety of our worldly possessions cross-country, about $1700. All told, our moving expenses for physically moving our stuff alone were about **$3000**.
  - o One more thing. Because our beloved couch did not fit in our pods, we had to sacrifice it and buy a new one in Pittsburgh. Add another **$1000**.
  - o Thus, it cost us **$7900 total** to move for fellowship.
  - o If a person chose to go high end and fly, ship their car and hire professional full-service movers, it would cost at least $10,000.
  - o Average of our route and the full-service price tag: **total of $8950**.
- **Fellowship program state licensing fees**
  - o As a fellow, you may or may not be reimbursed for state licensing fees. Arun's institution did happen to cover the cost.
  - o Some fellows do not have attending physician privileges during fellowship, and therefore do not pay licensing fees at the attending level.

- o Let's take Washington state as an example. After residency, the fees rise and fall under the "Physician and Surgeon (MD)" category. There is a **$491** application fee, then **$657** for a two-year renewal and **$60** for a certification of license, plus **$15** for each duplicate license.
- o Let's assume the general cost of licensing (which will vary by state) is **$1000 total**.
- **Medical board exam test prep courses and materials**
  - o Physicians study for and take board exams based on their specialty during their fellowship or after finishing residency. Board exams are the final "certification" step in training and must also be maintained throughout a physician's career.
  - o Of course, the pressure to succeed is high. For the field of Otolaryngology, the Osler Institute is the most popular choice for board preparation. Osler offers several study aids, including: in-person lecture ($920 for residents or fellows), home study audio guide ($475), board review quick hit guide ($99), and clinical case studies for the oral exam ($100) (The Osler Institute, 2016).
  - o Arun had a very busy fellowship year full of surgery, preparing for the birth of our daughter, and then learning how to be a dad—so he didn't have as much time to study as he would have liked. We paid $99 for online practice questions.
  - o Let's assume most people would go middle of the road and purchase the home study audio guide for **$475**, the quick hit guide for **$99**, and the oral exam case studies for **$100**. **Total: $674**.
- **Medical board exam fees**
  - o The board exam consists of two parts: computer-based testing at an approved testing center in the fall, and then (if the written exam is passed) an oral, in-person exam in the spring.
  - o This will vary by specialty, but the fees for the Otolaryngology board exam are **$3,580**. If you fail the written exam, tough luck—you must wait to take it again next year and there are certainly no refunds. Candidates who pass the written exam then get three consecutive chances to pass the oral exam (American Board of Otolaryngology, 2017).
  - o **Total: $3,580.**
- **Sitting for in-person oral exam for medical boards: travel expenses**

- If you pass the written exam, you need to get yourself to the in-person oral exam. For Arun, that meant traveling from Pittsburgh to Chicago.
- For most people, this generally involves round-trip airfare (his was $326), and a stay at the hotel where the exam is being given, usually one to two nights depending on the distance you have traveled (his was one night at $145). It may or may not require a rental car and/or taxi services.
- Let's assume that the average candidate spends **$400** on airfare, **$300** on a two-night hotel stay, and **$100** on car transport (either taxi or rental). **Total: $800.**

- **Maintenance of board certification**
  - There is an annual fee for maintaining board certification once you pass. For Otolaryngology, that fee is **$310** (American Board of Otolaryngology, 2017). This may or may not be reimbursed once the physician starts a full-time job.
  - Let's just include the first-year **total: $310**.

- **Professional association membership fees**
  - As working professionals, physicians generally belong to a handful of professional associations. Arun belongs to the American Academy of Otolaryngology—Head and Neck Surgery (**$890** annual dues) and American Head and Neck Society (**$400** annual dues).
  - Arun is fortunate to have these dues reimbursed by his employer. Let's assume most people would have the same benefit.
  - **Total: $0.**

- **A million and one things not included**
  - Not included: Lost income from several years of training (medical school, residency, fellowship), gallons and gallons of coffee required for survival, psychiatric bill to cope with stress of being a surgeon, and Match.com membership to meet a sugar mama.
  - While many of Arun's college buddies who had studied engineering and business graduated and immediately started earning six figures, Arun was still many years away from even a mediocre paycheck.
  - Lost income is significant, especially for surgeons. We're talking about millions of dollars here, easily. There is also a huge amount money lost in interest on retirement savings. I'll put it this way: in just a few months as an attending physician, Arun

accrued the same balance on his 401K as he did over six grueling years as a resident.

Have you skipped ahead to the final tally? The very length of this chapter should have been your first clue that this was not going to be cheap. At the end of the day, **it costs approximately $691,554 to become a surgeon in America**, and the price tag continues to escalate.

Memoirs of a Surgeon's Wife, by Megan Sharma

FREE PENS AND OTHER LUXURIES

Becoming a surgeon is not all financial strain and drain. The most notable benefits of residency are training related: subsidized research time, hands-on courses in surgical technique, industry conferences, and other national training events—all for free or with heavy discounts.

But wait, there's more! Act now and you can also receive:
- Conference SWAG: pens, notepads, and of course: the compulsory super cheap polyester conference messenger bag
- Nasal irrigation kits
- The hero of cold season: nasal decongestant spray

Who could resist such tempting treats?

Memoirs of a Surgeon's Wife, by Megan Sharma

PATIENCE AND PATIENTS AND THE ABUNDANCE OF BOTH

Let's consider volume for a moment. Doctors see a lot of patients, no doubt, but exactly how many?

Arun says that the average ENT resident sees about 20 patients per week. Multiply this by 50 weeks per year, and you get 1,000 patients seen each year. Arun's residency was six years long (minus one year of research), so he saw approximately 5,000 patients during his residency.

As far as surgeries during ENT residency, Arun estimates that he did many hundreds, if not over a thousand surgeries.

As an attending, Arun sees even more patients. In an academic setting with his time split between surgery, clinic, research and teaching residents and medical students, Arun sees 30-50 patients per week. Average is 40 patients per week. Multiply that by 47 weeks and you have 1,880 patients seen by Dr. Sharma annually.

Can you imagine?

There is no way to quantify this, but just think, how many of these patients...

...are grateful to see the doctor?

...have no medical problem whatsoever?

Memoirs of a Surgeon's Wife, by Megan Sharma

...are looking for an excuse to take some time off work without eating up vacation days?

...smell weird?

...only want prescription drugs?

...are genuinely concerned about their health?

...don't know why they are seeing the doctor today (either forgot or don't understand)?

...were referred by a well-meaning colleague but have no business in that waiting room?

...watched a medical show on TV and have already diagnosed themselves?

...are lonely and just need a chat?

...will never actually follow the wise advice given?

Fun game, right?

Memoirs of a Surgeon's Wife, by Megan Sharma

SLEEP PATTERNS

The sleep patterns of a surgical resident are interesting, indeed.

Predictably, hours of uninterrupted slumber are few and far between. Between late nights on call and early mornings spent frantically studying anatomy in preparation for surgery, it's no wonder that our couch became synonymous with our bed.

Might I be so bold as to advise others pursuing a career in medicine and their loved ones to invest in a decent quality couch? Forget a piece of crap starter couch from Ikea, or, heaven forbid, a secondhand futon. A couch with reclinable seats is also recommended. Why? Well...let's just say that sometimes the distance between the couch and the bed is symbolically greater than crossing the Grand Canyon.

During Arun's residency, it became nearly impossible for us to watch an entire movie together without him falling asleep before the credit roll. This irritated me to no end. Do I shake him awake? Pause the movie? Let him sleep and miss it? Argh. Can't win.

This wasn't limited to the confines of our condo, unfortunately. It happened at social gatherings. Our friends will never forget the time that Arun fell asleep during our weekly "Dexter" watching party. Thankfully, they were not offended.

The moral of the story: if you are a person who requires a lot of sleep to function (like me), do not become a surgeon. You'll thank me later.

Memoirs of a Surgeon's Wife, by Megan Sharma

BURNOUT

What does burning out mean? Does it mean that we go down in a fiery passion, perhaps even in a blaze of glory? Does it mean that the embers of our soul are slowly dying and fading away? Or have we finally exhausted all remnants of our will to care?

A wise friend in medicine told me, "you can't burn out if you never care." Regardless, the result is the same: the curtain closes and we move on, or we somehow find the drive to keep on going.

Burnout can happen to anyone, at any time, but it is most certainly linked to stress and high expectations. It sucks our energy and our joy. We may be able to go through the motions, but usually not more than that.

It is not uncommon during medical school or residency to witness burnout. People realize that the demands are too much, this isn't what they want, this isn't their priority in life.

There were a few cases of program dropouts or even people being let go among Arun's fellow trainees. It was rare, but it did happen.

I am going out on a limb to say that I don't think these people are failures. I think that something didn't click, it wasn't the right timing, the environment was poisonous, or it wasn't their true calling. Just like how relationships that seem so sunny and hopeful in the beginning don't always pan out.

Burnout isn't limited to trainees—it happens in the professional world, too.

Memoirs of a Surgeon's Wife, by Megan Sharma

The Mayo Clinic conducted a study "to evaluate the impact of organizational leadership on the professional satisfaction and burnout of individual physicians working for a large health care organization." (Tait D. Shanafelt M. G., 2015) By surveying physicians and scientists working for a large health care organization, the investigators found a strong correlation between physician satisfaction and supervisor leadership scores. The likelihood of burnout also decreased as the composite leadership score increased.

In plain English: when you like and admire the leadership qualities of your superiors, you are more likely to be satisfied with your job and less likely to burn out.

The Mayo Clinic also examined the "relationship between clerical burden and characteristics of the electronic environment with physician burnout and professional satisfaction." (Tait D. Shanafelt M. L., 2016) Oooh, juicy!

"Physicians across all specialties in the United States were surveyed between August and October 2014. Physicians provided information regarding use of electronic health records (EHRs), computerized physician order entry (CPOE), and electronic patient portals. Burnout was measured using validated metrics." (Tait D. Shanafelt M. L., 2016)

What did they find? Physician satisfaction with their EHRs and CPOE was "generally low." "Physicians who used EHRs and CPOE were less satisfied with the amount of time spent on clerical tasks and were at higher risk for professional burnout." (Tait D. Shanafelt M. L., 2016)

The analysis was adjusted for age, sex, specialty, practice setting, and hours worked per week—so we're not just talking about older physicians who prefer doing everything on paper.

What about medical/surgical specialty? Does that impact the potential for burnout?

Funny you should ask. One of Arun's residency colleagues, Dr. Justin S. Golub, studied that very question in the context of their shared specialty: Otolaryngology—Head and Neck Surgery. Dr. Golub worked with his mentor, Dr. Michael Johns III, to carry out Dr. Johns' vision.

Memoirs of a Surgeon's Wife, by Megan Sharma

As a fourth-year medical student at Emory University School of Medicine, Dr. Golub studied burnout in what would later become his 'tribe," Otolaryngology—Head and Neck Surgery residents. For brevity, let's call them "Oto" residents.

Dr. Golub employed the Maslach Burnout inventory (Maslach, 1996), which defines burnout as "a high degree of emotional exhaustion, a high degree of depersonalization, and a low sense of personal accomplishment. *Emotional exhaustion is the feeling of being emotionally overextended and fatigued by one's work. Depersonalization is the adoption of a callous or dehumanized perception of others.* Often, emotional exhaustion and the depletion of emotional resources can lead to depersonalization. Low *personal accomplishment* is the feeling of dissatisfaction with one's work-related achievements." (Justin S. Golub P. S., 2007)

My translation: feeling drained to the core, disconnected from the people around you, and intensely disappointed with yourself.

This was the first national-scale study on the topic of burnout worldwide. It's important because resident burnout can result in "poor quality of patient care, decreased productivity, and personal dysfunction." (Justin S. Golub P. S., 2007) We'll talk more about what can result from personal dysfunction later in this chapter.

Dr. Golub et al. found through their national survey of Oto residents that burnout was "strikingly prevalent," "with 86 percent of residents expressing either moderate (76 percent) or high levels of burnout (10 percent)." (Justin S. Golub P. S., 2007) The strongest contributing factor was work hours.

Interestingly, although perhaps not surprisingly, as the public has little sympathy for the "plight" of physicians in America, little attention has been drawn to this issue until more recent years. Per the study, "our data agree with cited evidence that, among residents, burnout is likely more prevalent than depression or substance abuse, two subjects that gain far more attention in the workplace." (Justin S. Golub P. S., 2007)

Well, this is all a big downer, isn't it? What can we do to exact change in the right direction?

The study authors say, "The disturbingly high prevalence of burnout should serve as a wake-up call to residency directors, not only in otolaryngology, but in all specialties. Adherence to the [sic] ACGME 80-hour workweek guidelines, introduction of more control and flexibility into curricula, establishment of support groups for residents and spouses, and consideration of reasonable grievances regarding professional stressors represent several ways the epidemic of burnout may be contained and treated." (Justin S. Golub P. S., 2007)

Dr. Golub went on to study burnout among Oto academic faculty. He found that "burnout was prevalent among U.S. academic otolaryngologists, although levels were lower than those of Otolaryngology chairs and residents. Modification of risk factors, such as allowing sufficient faculty time for research and administrative activities, should be undertaken to curb the development of burnout and its deleterious sequelae." (Justin S. Golub, Michael M. Johns, Paul S. Weiss, & Atul K. Ramesh, 2008)

In the face of burnout, I would encourage anyone to stop, think, evaluate: what is it that I want out of life? Can I see myself doing this for the next few decades? What if my children want to follow in my professional footsteps—will I welcome them with open arms, or warn them against it?

And, finally, how can I change things for the better?

Burnout can have even more devastating results. Each year in the United States, roughly 300-400 physicians die by suicide (American Foundation for Suicide Prevention, 2016). A doctor a day, if you will—and probably more, due to inaccurate cause of death reporting and coding, likely by sympathetic colleagues in the morgue (Louise B Andrew, 2016).

Furthermore, suicide deaths are 250-400 percent higher among female physicians when compared to females in other professions (American Foundation for Suicide Prevention, 2016). "Of all occupations and professions, the medical profession consistently hovers near the top of occupations with the highest risk of death by suicide." (Louise B Andrew, 2016)

The loss of any life is tragic, but these numbers are more significant than they initially seem. The number of physician suicide deaths each year is equivalent to the size of an entire medical school class (Louise B Andrew, 2016). Poof—gone.

Of course, the impact to the deceased's family, friends and colleagues is monumental. Patients are also affected. "Given that a typical doctor has about 2,300 patients under his or her care, that means more than a million Americans will lose a physician to suicide this year." (Wible, 2014)

Memoirs of a Surgeon's Wife, by Megan Sharma

This is not a new problem. "It has been known for more than 150 years that physicians have an increased propensity to die by suicide." (Louise B Andrew, 2016) Yet, it is a problem that has only surfaced in the American media in recent years.

Why is that? And why are so many doctors taking their own lives with such brutal accuracy, aided by their expert knowledge of the human body?

A quick Google search is enough to get a basic grasp on what's happening, through headlines like "American Doctors Are Killing Themselves and No One Is Talking About It," and "Physicians have the highest suicide rate of any profession. So why haven't you heard about it?"

Getting down to brass tacks on the forces behind physician suicide is less complicated than you might think. Suicide is preventable.

"In every population, suicide is almost invariably the result of untreated or inadequately treated depression or other mental illness that may or may not include substance or alcohol abuse, coupled with knowledge of and access to lethal means." (Gagné P, 2011)

Here's another chilling statistic: medical students have rates of depression 15 to 30 percent higher than the general population. Depression is a major risk factor in physician suicide (American Foundation for Suicide Prevention, 2016).

Depression, bipolar disorder, alcoholism, and substance abuse are the usual suspects. There is a prevailing social stigma associated with these afflictions in almost every culture around the world—so asking for and receiving lifesaving help is not only difficult, it may be nearly impossible. But does this tell the whole story?

There are other factors in play. Day-to-day pressures including a never-ending work day, jabs with insurance companies, the necessity of keeping up with current medical research and education, mountains of personal debt, increasing government regulations and the ensuing administrative burden, and the ever-present fear of legal action.

Dr. Pamela Wible, an internal medicine doctor in Eugene, Oregon practicing for more than 20 years, offers her thoughts on why "so many healers are harming themselves": "We see far too much pain; to ask for help is considered a weakness; to visit a psychiatrist can be professional suicide, meaning that we risk loss of license

Memoirs of a Surgeon's Wife, by Megan Sharma

and hospital privileges, not to mention wariness from patients if our emotional distress becomes known." (Wible, 2014)

The irony is that "although physicians seem to have generally heeded their own advice about avoiding smoking and other common risk factors for early mortality, they are decidedly reluctant to address depression, a significant cause of morbidity and mortality that disproportionately affects them." (Louise B Andrew, 2016)

For many, asking for help simply isn't an option. "A survey of American surgeons revealed that although 1 in 16 had experienced suicidal ideation in the past 12 months, only 26 percent of those with suicidal ideation had sought psychiatric or psychologic help." (Shanafelt TD, 2011) "There was a strong correlation between depressive symptoms, as well as indicators of burnout, with the incidence of suicidal ideation." (Louise B Andrew, 2016)

And why not nip the problem in the bud? "More than 60 percent of those with suicidal ideation indicated they were reluctant to seek help due to concern that it could affect their medical license." (Shanafelt TD, 2011)

What happens next? "An obstetrician is found dead in his bathtub; gunshot wound to the head. An anesthesiologist dies of an overdose in a hospital closet. A family doctor is hit by a train. An internist at a medical conference jumps from his hotel balcony to his death. All true stories." (Wible, 2014)

There is more that we can do. We can face the statistics head on, instead of sweeping them under the rug. We can stop the cycle of teaching medical students, residents and fellows that keeping a stiff upper lip is more important than maintaining mental and emotional health. We must stop propagating the myth that physicians are infallible and accept the reality that we are all very much human. We can stop "blaming and shaming," as Dr. Wible advises. We can stop telling doctors that they should be happy because of the amount of money they make or will someday make. We can listen and take seriously the concerns and stresses of medical trainees and professionals. We can say something when we notice a colleague faltering, speaking a kind word rather than silencing our intuition and shrinking from an awkward situation. We can put in place resources, ideally anonymous, that give doctors a safe place to call for help—like a depression, substance abuse, and suicide hotline. We can start education and awareness early on—why not build it into medical school training? We can help physicians in their professional lives by providing continuing medical education on dealing with stress and death on the job.

Memoirs of a Surgeon's Wife, by Megan Sharma

And we can stop punishing those who somehow gather the courage and humility to ask for help with disdain, distrust, and threats to professional and personal livelihood.

The worst thing we can do is turn our backs and close our hearts to the suffering of others.

Memoirs of a Surgeon's Wife, by Megan Sharma

PUT DOWN THE PHAD THAI

There are more than 3,000 restaurants in Seattle, according to TripAdvisor. It's one of the most restaurant-dense cities in the country. We knew this to be true because there were a few dozen restaurants within walking distance of our condo, and we were not hurting for good grub.

When you're "eating healthy," on the other hand, takeout is the last thing you need. You need to put down the phad thai and drag your jiggly peanut sauce ass to the grocery store for some SALAD.

An abundance of walkable restaurants and a walk score of 98/100, we had. What we lacked was a decent grocery store that we didn't have to fight unreasonable traffic to get to.

Our primary challenge, although seemingly unrelated, was the fact that as a resident Arun was on call an average of twice a week. Yet, we still had to eat approximately three times a day (negotiable for Arun, but not for me!).

This meant that most the time, unless it was a weekend and Arun was not working, the grocery shopping fell to me, the non-doctor with a regular job.

Challenge #2: no parking spot. Early in our relationship, I didn't have a parking spot in our condo building, which meant that I had to chance it with street parking and pay a meter. There wasn't even a surface level paid lot that I could use nearby. So, when I did venture out on a grocery shopping excursion, I had to pray that the parking gods would smile upon me. Then, I would have to schlep bags and bags of groceries generally down the block and across the street, hope the door man would just buzz me in for god's sake, keep it together and operate an elevator, and finally unlock the condo door and dump everything inside. There were often multiple trips to and from the car. And I got rained on quite a bit, because—Seattle.

After complaining about this for too long, I rented a parking spot in the building, which blessedly kept wheeled carts in the garage elevator bay to help people with too much stuff to carry.

We also tried Amazon Fresh, a grocery delivery service, which at the time was only available in Seattle. It was convenient, but pricey and a little lackluster. Not as appealing as food shopping with your eyes and with your stomach in person.

Challenge #3: wheels go buh-bye. After losing my parking spot in the building for the third or fourth time with essentially no notice and nowhere else to park it, I'd had enough. I decided to get rid of the damn car. I worked a mile away, in fact—I could walk! Why had I been so lazy in the first place? Plus, we still had Arun's car and a Zipcar station right next to our building. That was all well and good, until Arun was on call and I had no ride. I did this for a whole year and a half, in fact. It was a humbling experience. I felt like a teenager again, bumming a ride with my friends to go see a movie.

I have it good here in central Illinois, now. We have a walk score of zero but my Acura is a breeze to drive and I don't mind stopping at the grocery store whenever I feel like it.

At least I'll be able to tell my grandchildren one day that humans can endure without cars—though it ain't always easy.

Memoirs of a Surgeon's Wife, by Megan Sharma

IT'S WORTH NOTING: YOUR DOCTOR IS A HUMAN BEING

D octor oh doctor
> Gimme the news I got a
> Pager never rests

Whether you know it or not, your doctor has made many a sacrifice for you and your overall well-being.

I can tell you with absolute certainty that your personal cornucopia of doctors has:

- Stayed up all night for you (for example, performing an emergency surgery)
- Checked on your status while at home watching TV
- Secretly emailed/texted/called a colleague while out with friends or significant others to make sure your plan of care was communicated effectively
- Cried or worried over you—your tragedy does not fall on deaf ears
- Missed a social event because of you
- Gone without eating or drinking for countless hours while treating you
- Been inspired by your story

Memoirs of a Surgeon's Wife, by Megan Sharma

- Delayed an airport trip (likely for a well-deserved vacation) on your account
- Talked about you (anonymously) in a medical journal or at a conference—you're just that interesting!
- Interrupted sex to answer a page on your behalf
- Made the near impossible possible for you, like getting you into that stellar assisted living facility on short notice
- Wondered whether they did everything they could for you
- Hoped the very best for you
- Missed out on being home for the holidays so they could be there for you
- Been humbled by your outlook on life, and by your kindness

It helps to remember on occasion that the people we deal with in our lives are exactly that: people with their own feelings, dreams and insecurities. Doctors serve willingly and, in most cases, genuinely care for their patients.

Memoirs of a Surgeon's Wife, by Megan Sharma

ON BECOMING A SUGAR MAMA

During the Hindu portion of our wedding ceremony, my father-in-law, Prabhakar, who was performing the ceremony, built in a few helpful tips for my husband-to-be. "Keep her happy. Always take her to the Nordstrom," he implored with a mischievous chortle. At the time Prabhakar was blissfully unaware of two facts: 1) next to nothing could keep me from "the Nordstrom," and 2) With Arun's salary as a resident, we should be shopping exclusively at Walmart and on special occasions, perhaps, at Nordstrom Rack.

Let's just say that Arun is blessed to have found his sugar mama early in his residency career.

Arun did have some "tried and true" money-saving techniques that only a single dude would employ:
- Rather than wasting money on frivolous wine glasses, we drank vino from tall water glasses. Classy.
- Wearing t-shirts from high school that bore a stunning resemblance to Swiss cheese and adamantly refusing to get rid of them.
- Getting his hair cut exclusively at Great Clips. I tolerated this for far too long, even though he would often come home with slightly uneven sideburns or a duly unkempt neckline. "But it only costs $12!" he would exclaim. Yeah, and they don't even shampoo your hair, like any civilized salon would. He always had to shower after a haircut because of all the little gross hairs everywhere. The final straw was one evening when he came home fresh from the Great Clips. I took one look at the back of his head and gasped. There was literally a line in the middle of his head where the

"stylist" (hack artist) had trimmed/shaved only the bottom third of his head. The top 2/3 looked the same length as when he left the house. He didn't even bother to look in the mirror at the "salon," because they didn't offer. OMG! It was a true hair emergency. He could not go out in public looking like that, never mind to work the next day. So, we paid a visit to a friend who does hair and he, bless his soul, managed to salvage the wreckage of Arun's traumatized follicles. Thank you, Rah! You are a miracle worker! Since that day, I have enacted a lifetime ban on Great Clips, and on this I will not waver.

Otherwise, he was a pretty normal and reasonable bachelor when I met him. But wealthy, he was not.

I was under the false impression that all doctors made a lot of money, like many people. It didn't occur to me that as a resident, you are still considered a student, and are therefore earning what amounts to a student salary.

When Arun began his six-year residency in 2008, the mean actual stipend for first-year residents and fellows in the U.S. was $46,245 (AAMC, 2016). Interestingly, back in 1968 when this survey was first conducted by the AAMC, the same figure was $6,200.

As you move through residency, the salary does increase, veerrrryyyyy sloowwwwlllyyyyy.

For example, the mean actual stipend increase from the first post-MD year in 2012-2013 to the second-year in 2014 was $2,739, or 5.4 percent (AAMC, 2016).

By the 6th post-MD year (at the end of my husband's residency), the mean actual stipend was $61,493 (AAMC, 2016).

Of course, this doesn't account for the cost of living in an expensive city like Seattle. Residents are not provided housing or any other benefits besides their stipend/salary—they are on their own. And many residents are also drowning in medical school debt upwards of $100,000.

Residents are required to reside within a reasonable distance of the hospital(s) at which they work, generally within a 15 to 20-minute drive, at most. Since most hospitals with residency programs are in city centers, this ups the price of housing. Residents can't get away with living in the middle of nowhere for dirt cheap.

Per the US Census Bureau, the median value of owner-occupied housing units in the city of Seattle from 2010-2014 was $437,400. For the same four years, the median selected monthly owner costs, with a mortgage, were $2307.00 (US Census Bureau, 2016). That is consistent with our mortgage and HOA fees in the heart of the city for those years. We paid a bit more.

Tell me, then...how is a resident who earns around $50,000 annually supposed to afford a $2500 mortgage? That's 60 percent of their gross salary. Answer: they can't. That's what parents and sugar mamas/daddies are for.

Things wouldn't be much easier if Arun had chosen to rent rather than buy. The median gross rent for 2010-2014 was $1,131 (US Census Bureau, 2016). That price would have gotten you a 400-square foot studio in the downtown Seattle area, probably in some shady digs next to the neighborhood drug dealer. Rent prices have only skyrocketed since we moved in 2014.

It's not just the housing. Everything in Seattle is more expensive than say, the Midwest. Groceries. Gas. Restaurants. Oil changes. Forbes says that Seattle and surrounding areas (including Bellevue and Everett) are 21.3 percent above the national average for cost of living (Forbes, 2016).

And consider these professions that earn more money than the average medical resident (who has already earned an M.D.) (Salary.com, 2016):
- Bingo Manager: $56,593
- Elevator Inspector: $59,495
- Soil Conservationist: $62,228
- Locomotive Engineer: $63,620
- Clinical Ethicist: $66,966
- Prosthetist/Orthotist: $67,938
- Enterostomal Therapist: $74,639. The description of this job is interesting. "An enterostomy is an operation in which the surgeon cuts a passage into the patient's small intestine, through the abdomen. The newly created opening allows for the drainage of fecal matter or to insert a feeding tube. This procedure is used mostly in emergency cases of severe abdomen wounds and diseases such as certain types of cancer and Crohn's disease. The enterostomal therapist must not only care for the stoma post-surgery, but also educate patients on how to properly care for it. Patients

cannot leave the hospital until they know how to properly care for themselves after the surgery, and until they learn, enterostomal therapists are charged with cleaning and sanitizing the stoma for them." What I find most fascinating is that the Enterostomal Therapist who is quite literally helping the patient "keep their shit together" is earning more money than the General Surgery resident who is likely performing the surgery (under the direct supervision of the attending General Surgeon).

It's even more outrageous to think in terms of an hourly wage. Residents are prohibited from working an average of more than 80 hours per week. Assuming we are working with a $50,000 salary, that equates to about $12 per hour. In 2015, the city of Seattle (where Arun worked as a resident) passed a minimum wage ordinance that will gradually increase the minimum wage to $15 per hour (Seattle.gov, 2016). This means that Seattle-based residents are, in effect, earning less than the citywide minimum wage.

The moral of the story is this: it's about time that we started paying residents and fellows a fair wage that is in line with the regional cost of living at their institution.

Not everyone can have their very own IT Corporate Communications sugar mama/daddy, after all. We are a rare and wonderful breed of awesome.

Memoirs of a Surgeon's Wife, by Megan Sharma

12-HOUR SURGERIES AND DENYING ESSENTIAL BODILY FUNCTIONS

Let's get one thing straight: I cannot accomplish anything when I am hungry. The mere idea of food pervades my every sense and thought and prevents me from achieving any real form of productivity. I can't write when I'm hungry, I can't respond to email when I am hungry, I can't even shop for rain boots on Zappos when I am hungry. The situation must be *dealt with* in the form of a protein bar or a delightfully tangy yogurt before the ordinary pace of life may proceed.

To me, as an active and frequent consumer of nutritional substance, it's pretty mind-boggling to imagine a 12-hour fast that represents only 75 percent of an average work day, never mind spending this 12 hours on my feet, in active concentration, trying not to kill someone while removing CANCER from their body.

Are you kidding me???

That's the reality of being a surgeon. While not all surgeries last 12 hours, a series of several shorter surgeries (three to five hours each) can easily consume an entire day. Add clinic patients to the mix and the fact that emails and pages never stop, and you've got one self-denying human robot.

Memoirs of a Surgeon's Wife, by Megan Sharma

Not only do surgeons regularly deny themselves (at a minimum) lunch and dinner at remotely appropriate times, they also categorically abandon the idea of hydration.

What goes in must come out, right?

My bladder could not be more undisciplined, as my friends and family will readily tell you. Expect multiple disruptions if you choose to shop a Black Friday sale with me, or road trip in excess of 60 minutes.

It makes me feel guilty that at my ordinary nine-to-five-er, I always kept at least two beverages at my desk: water and an Americano before 11:00 a.m., water and black tea from 11:00 a.m.-1:00 p.m., and water and Diet Coke or Pepsi from 1:00 p.m. onward. Naturally curious minds may intuit the results of this one-woman liquid refreshment parade: I had to pee, constantly!

It would astound me to have peed any less than once every hour while on the job.

So, the next time you pop the top on that third Mountain Dew of the work day, think of the surgeons in your local hospital, hoping to sweat out the urge to pee, never being offered a bathroom break.

Memoirs of a Surgeon's Wife, by Megan Sharma

WHEN MEDICINE MEETS MEDICINE

What happens when you work exceptionally long hours at the hospital, have no free time, and little energy to date outside the workplace? Medicine meets medicine!

Nearly 40 percent of physicians are likely to marry another physician or health care professional, according to the 2014 Work/Life Profiles of Today's U.S. Physician released by AMA Insurance (AMA Insurance, 2016).

I can see it. Your day gets a little brighter when that cute doctor makes her rounds. Before you know it, you're finding excuses to run into her, asking her out to coffee, and then treasuring your "secret" relationship with knowing grins.

If the relationship gets serious, there are many challenges ahead. Especially if you are both doctors, but for any medical relationship, there are all too many opportunities for space to come between you. Namely: medical school, residency, fellowship, and career choices.

At these stages, there is the potential to pick up and move, and that's difficult if one person is already settled in a job and city.

Thankfully, there is hope: couples can apply to the same medical school, residency, and fellowship. The caveat is that it's far more competitive to secure two spots at the same institution than it is for an individual. And to get to the point of matching with a program, the couple must agree on how they rank each institution and present a united front.

Memoirs of a Surgeon's Wife, by Megan Sharma

There are no guarantees. It is all or nothing. If a couple doesn't match into residency or fellowship together, their applications cannot be processed separately to find a possible match for each individual.

What if the couple is at different points in their training and career? This happens all the time. For example, one person is graduating from medical school before the other. You cannot apply to match together. What to do in that situation? Does the graduate tack on another degree (and even more debt), or find some sort of temporary job in the meantime? Or do they continue down the line and leave their loved one (temporarily) behind, praying that the time will go by quickly?

We have known committed and married couples who have lived in different cities/states for a year or more to further their careers. That's something I cannot imagine doing, because my husband and I have been like Indian/American conjoined twins ever since the day we met.

There are so many choices to be made. But it's not like a "Choose your Own Adventure" book where you can skip ahead to see if you will like the result.

With two doctors in the house, whose career takes priority? The reality of life is that something's gotta give. Both careers were equally hard fought. Both people have unique and valuable skills. Both are passionate about what they do. Both deserve to follow their dreams. But in the end, who compromises? Because somebody must.

In the absence of compromise "home" can become nothing more than a crash pad full of greasy old takeout boxes, unattended dirty laundry, and searingly empty white walls.

If children are in the picture, child care must revolve around two hectic physician schedules and must be reliable, no matter what.

Arun and I count ourselves lucky that we didn't have to face the same hurdles as those faced by double doctor couples. My career has always been more flexible. Our experience combining two lives with completely different career trajectories has been overwhelmingly positive, but we do struggle just like everyone else.

Memoirs of a Surgeon's Wife, by Megan Sharma

Considering all they are up against, we have the utmost respect for medical couples and admire their ability to keep their relationships front and center amidst a constant tug-of-war for time and energy. Keep fighting the good fight, ya'll!

Memoirs of a Surgeon's Wife, by Megan Sharma

THE OTHER SHOE

It finally happened: the day my husband wore two different shoes to work. May 21, 2014. We hoped this day would never come, but fate had other designs.

Arun had been on call two nights prior. Call nights had been particularly painful as of late, since crashing with my parents 25 miles outside the city meant that he had to sleep at the hospital overnight in decidedly un-luxurious accommodations.

It was a largely sleepless night, involving an emergency slash trach and buckets of blood. An hour and a half total snooze time.

Then, the next day, he had an incredibly complex surgery that didn't end until 10:36 p.m. Catching up on a day's worth of work since he'd been in surgery, I didn't see him until after midnight. And he was the walking dead, as expected.

The next morning, he woke around 4:00, as usual, kissed me, and headed to work.

A few hours later, Arun called me in between hospitals and gave me the news: he was wearing one brown dress shoe and one black dress shoe, a difference imperceptible in the dark of our borrowed bedroom. Shockingly comfortable, he said.

Of course, this happened to fall on the day of his weekly conference when every attending physician and resident in the program is present. The residents mocked him mercilessly, taking photos like paparazzi amid his tragedy.

Even worse, he had made fun of a former resident a few years ago, for this very same offense.

Memoirs of a Surgeon's Wife, by Megan Sharma

I told him that his clinic patients surely would be entertained, but they didn't utter a word.

Only time will tell the long-term impacts of this day. For now, we both just want to say, we're sorry for making fun of you before, Nikki! Karma, right?

Memoirs of a Surgeon's Wife, by Megan Sharma

VACATION, ALL I EVER WANTED. VACATION, HAD TO GET AWAY.

In the Sharma family, we stack up vacations like dominos. If we don't have at least one or two to look forward to, it's game over!

It was no different during Arun's residency, although our budget was humbler.

I prefer international vacations because they are the key to truly disconnecting from work. Sorry, we won't have phone or email! Deal with it! That worked until recently, when T-Mobile decided to let us use our Wi-Fi and data internationally. Then there was the invention of WhatsApp, which lets us make international calls for free. Le sigh.

But back in the day, traveling abroad, even to Mexico or Canada, meant that work didn't stow away with either of us. And that was a welcome retreat.

Arun's intern year, his first year of residency, was the worst. His vacation schedule was set for him and he had absolutely no control over when it would take place. He ended up with two weeks of vacation very close together and then waiting for what seemed like an eternity for his final week off.

During residency Arun had three weeks of vacation per year like a lot of Americans, with a few key differences:
- Senior residents' vacation schedules always take precedent.

Memoirs of a Surgeon's Wife, by Megan Sharma

- During the months of June and July, every year, no one can take a single vacation day. The reason is that all new residents begin on July 1, nationwide. So, it's a very busy time and a time of transition. If you have a wedding or graduation to attend, you are out of luck. As a result, Arun missed the weddings of a cousin and a close friend.
- The vacation must be taken in a consecutive week. It cannot be broken up into individual days (forget about creating a bunch of long weekends).
- There is no guarantee that you will not be stuck on call for at least one weekend before or after your vacation.
- Friday night red eyes are not possible—surgery can (and typically does) run late. Arun inevitably ends up working very late the night before we are to leave for vacation, even now. We call it the night before vacation curse.

One of our most memorable trips together was also our first plane trip and international getaway as a pair, a few months into our relationship.

We traveled to Puerto Vallarta, Mexico to celebrate the end of Arun's intern year in 2009. All-inclusive resort, pristine beach, blessedly relaxing. The locals kept mistaking Arun for being Mexican, even though he could barely say "hola."

Toward the end of our vacation, Arun wanted to do something special for me. He arranged a dinner at one of the best restaurants in old town, La Palapa, which was a 45-minute cab ride from our resort.

We set off in a taxi on our romantic outing. Not far from our destination, a torrential downpour came out of nowhere. So much water fell from the skies that the "charming" cobblestone streets (with terrible water management systems) flooded immediately. There were literally rivers running down city streets and sidewalks. We later learned that this happens all the time – you just need to be careful to avoid it.

Our cab driver was less than adventurous and refused to take us all the way to the restaurant. The language barrier made it difficult to understand where the restaurant was. It seemed to be within a few blocks. This was before people traveled abroad with smart phones, so we couldn't just Google Map it.

It was a decision point: skulk back to the resort and bemoan the rain and our missed meal of magnificence or continue into the (slippery) unknown. We decided, YOLO! (That one is for you, Amar). We went for it.

Memoirs of a Surgeon's Wife, by Megan Sharma

We were both dressed up: Arun in khakis, new leather shoes and a dress shirt, and I in a dress and flat gladiator sandals, thank heavens.

We ran with only the faintest idea of where we were heading in coffee-colored rushing water that was up to a foot deep at times.

After only a few minutes, we were soaked to the bone. Lost and looking like drowned rats in resort wear, we stopped into a neighborhood bar to dry off a bit, and to drink more than a bit.

The bar's owner was Canadian and took pity on us. She gave us garbage bags as makeshift ponchos to protect us from the elements. After a couple of margaritas, we were okay with that!

On we slogged, with slightly better directions as our guide.

Eventually, two very determined, drenched patrons arrived at the upscale restaurant sporting designer garbage bags. The staff welcomed us and even provided towels for our comfort! It was a memorable night, indeed.

Memoirs of a Surgeon's Wife, by Megan Sharma

POWER NAPPING IN SURGERY

Is it possible to fall asleep during surgery? If it's possible to fall asleep while talking on the phone, watching Netflix, studying for an exam, or playing mini golf, then it is also possible to fall asleep while in surgery.

Whattttt????

I know, this sounds completely awful. But note that I said while *in surgery,* not while *operating.* There is a big difference, dahh-ling.

In the operating room, there are generally quite a few people present. The surgeon(s), of course. One or more residents. Perhaps a medical student. And the OR nursing staff. At other times, there might also be a student on an away rotation or a visitor from a different country. These individuals don't necessarily play an active role in the surgery. Too many surgeons in the kitchen, as they say.

Depending on the type of surgery, it can be a sideline sport. A person's sole endeavor during a six plus hour surgery might be to watch and learn. Or, to put some muscle into the game, they might be asked to retract (physically holding tissue to keep the surgical field exposed).

Surgery is not always as juicy as the latest celebrity scandal in US Weekly. And thus...the power nap is possible.

Although certainly not encouraged and extremely embarrassing when revealed, napping in the OR is a real thing.

Memoirs of a Surgeon's Wife, by Megan Sharma

THE BUSINESS OF HEALTH CARE

I can hear you yawning, dear reader. I know, I know—so much has already been written on the business of health care that I've already lost you. But hear me out. I'm not going to rehash the innumerable discussions of this topic already swirling around America. I'm not going to talk about The Affordable Care Act (Obamacare). I'm not going to propose a government-run health care system like the one in Canada. I'm not even going to villainize the insurance agencies and lawyers—well, not too much.

All I can do is tell you about a recent experience of my husband's and let you draw your own (extremely leading) conclusions.

Arun saw a patient in clinic who needed surgery. He needed robotic surgery, and it wasn't going to be cheap. The patient, unfortunately, was saddled with a low-cost insurance provider.

Almost immediately, the insurance company refused to allow the patient his surgery. Feeling the surgery was necessary for his patient, Arun set about navigating the process of connecting with the insurance company to explain why the patient's surgery should, in fact, be covered.

First, Arun was given a general 800 number to call. After spending an inordinate amount of time trying to decipher a secret path to a live person in the complex automated phone menu, Arun finally reached a live human being. Much to his dismay, that agent was in the wrong state. Then, he had to be transferred to the correct department in the correct state. Insert more hold time here.

Memoirs of a Surgeon's Wife, by Megan Sharma

Arun said the experience was very Comcast-esque. Comcast, by comparison, would have been a shining beacon of customer service.

When Arun reached the department for the correct state, they had no idea what he was talking about when he requested a "peer-to-peer," the specific words used by the insurance company representatives from the first state. It's self-explanatory and generally well known in the industry: Arun wanted to talk to one of the doctors at the insurance company with decision-making authority.

After explaining that a few times, Arun was told that he would need to leave his name, phone number, and a few dates and times that he was available to talk, and they would call him back. Not like he had patients to worry about, or anything. Meanwhile, the clock was ticking down the days until the patient's scheduled surgery.

After two days, Arun never received any contact from the insurance agency. Arun asked his clinical staff to hunt down a direct number for a physician within the insurance company, which they did. He called again. Still, a dead end. They never circled back to him.

In the end, the insurance company held firm in their refusal to cover the surgery for the patient. The surgery was canceled. And...now what? The patient is no better off than when Arun first met him and must wait 60-90 days to appeal the decision. Just so the insurance company can get a little bit richer.

That's the business of American health care today.

Memoirs of a Surgeon's Wife, by Megan Sharma

I HAD THOSE DEGREES PRINTED AT KINKO'S. JUST KIDDING. IT WAS FEDEX OFFICE.

Arun and I have a running joke that he had his multiple degrees and accolades printed at Kinko's (this shows you how far back the joke runs). Man, that sure would have been easier than the reality!

There are many times that we wonder if he spent the better part of his golden years working his booty off and studying like a madman just so that he could be an "expert" in the following:

- Carving turkey
- Cutting birthday cake
- Portioning lasagna
- Sawing through bone

Wait...that last one is something he does for work. That's legit.

Joking aside, it does get you thinking. How many people work in the field for which they studied? How many feel that their investments of time and money have paid off with a spectacular career? How many are working, period?

Per a 2014 survey by CareerBuilder, 45 percent of employed 2014 college graduates (from four-year institutions) are in jobs that don't require a degree.

Adding even more color to the picture, "Sixty-five percent of recent college grads are employed, four percent are in internships, and 31 percent are not working at all, although many in the latter group simply haven't started their job search or are already back in school to pursue a higher degree." (CareerBuilder, 2016)

The survey also indicated that among graduates currently working, 51 percent said their job is related to their college major (CareerBuilder, 2016). So, a coin toss, essentially. A coin toss that determines if graduates are doing what they set out to do with their college education.

There is some hope, thankfully. Says the survey, "health care and STEM (science, technology, engineering, and math) graduates are slightly more likely to be employed full-time than non-STEM graduates (40 percent vs. 34 percent)." (CareerBuilder, 2016)

Another 2016 survey commissioned by CareerBuilder revealed that there is a growing skill gap in the U.S., with demand for graduates with degrees in Computer and Information Sciences, Nursing, Pharmaceuticals, Human Resources, Engineering, and other fields, far outpacing supply (CareerBuilder, 2016). For example, there was an average of 242,884 nursing jobs in the U.S. that went unfilled each month between January 2015 and January 2016 (CareerBuilder, 2016).

What I take away from all this is that a bachelor's degree is expected for the professional working world. "Data from the Bureau of Labor Statistics shows that workers with no college experience are twice as likely to be unemployed than those with a bachelor's degree or higher." (CareerBuilder, 2016)

However, investing in a college education is not a guarantee that you will automatically land a job in your desired field.

If you are pursuing a more traditional or linear path like medicine or law, your chances are better. But it's still a gamble. You may still want to keep FedEx Office on your back burner.

Memoirs of a Surgeon's Wife, by Megan Sharma

YES, BOSS. WHATEVER YOU SAY, BOSS

Here is a story straight from my husband about an on-the-job experience during residency. Take it away, Arun!

I rode in a car with Joe* and Billy Bob* today (*names have been changed to protect privacy; two senior attending physicians). This is all true.

We were leaving a meeting and heading to another one in a different part of town. We took the elevators to get to the parking garage. Joe went the wrong way and we got stuck in a stairwell, so we then had to take an emergency exit and walk down the parking ramp.

Joe complained about having to drive his wife's car, "This car is a piece of shit. I don't understand why she likes it so much. It's her stupid car. I hate it."

Then, we couldn't get out of the parking garage because Joe didn't pay his parking ticket and there was no attendant.

Joe: "What the F***?? This is ridiculous. I have better things to do with my time. I have a conference call. Let's go guys, let's figure this out. Let's do something about this."

Billy Bob started calling the emergency security number in the garage. Meanwhile, Joe got out of his car and started lifting the parking gate, which was hilarious. Joe made Billy Bob and I lift the gate up completely so that he could drive out without paying. We then jumped into the car and sped away before security arrived.

Memoirs of a Surgeon's Wife, by Megan Sharma

While driving, Joe remembered that he was supposed to be on a conference call. First, he couldn't operate his phone, so Billy Bob and I did it for him. Then, Billy Bob joined the call and pretended to be Joe for a bit (which was ludicrous, considering Billy Bob and Joe sound nothing alike).

Finally, Joe got on the phone while driving erratically. He nearly got us t-boned twice and almost hit a pedestrian.

What a day. Not sure I will get into a car with Joe again.

Memoirs of a Surgeon's Wife, by Megan Sharma

I'M THROWING YOUR DAMN PAGER INTO THE OCEAN

Have you ever fantasized about destroying an electronic nemesis, such as a laptop, cell phone, or set of Rosetta Stone disks? Sure, you have. Let me tell you about the object of my evilest energy: the pager.

Firstly, a pager (Bellis, About.com History of Pagers and Beepers, 2013) is a "dedicated radio frequency device that allows the pager user to receive messages broadcast on a specific frequency over a special network of radio base stations." I feel the need to include this definition for those readers born after 1990.

Here's how it works: one person sends a message, usually by phone, to the pager of the other person. The person carrying the pager hears a loud beep or feels a vibration that lets them know they have a message, or page. Then, the receiver sees the phone number or text message on a tiny little pager screen. Et, voilà.

My husband uses a one-way pager, which means there is practically no limit to the number of pages he can receive (okay, that's a lie, it can store up to 19 at a time), but he cannot respond directly from the pager itself—he must call or track the person down like a bounty hunter.

And who do medical professionals and their loved ones the world over have to thank for this glorious invention? That would be a Mr. Al Gross, who patented the very first telephone pager that was used by the Jewish Hospital in New York starting

Memoirs of a Surgeon's Wife, by Megan Sharma

in 1950 (Bellis, 2013). This was not a widely available technology until it was approved by the FCC for public use in 1958.

Motorola was the brand that started it all in 1959 and even coined the name "pager." Two decades and some change later, there were 3.2 million pager users worldwide. By 1994, more than 61 million pagers were in use and pagers were popular for personal use (About.com History of Pagers and Beepers).

Today, hospitals use pagers for their reliability and simplicity in an environment where cell phone coverage is often weak. You will even find flashy red beepy pagers at The Cheesecake Factory, which lets salivating customers know that their table awaits.

For those of you who have not experienced the sound of a pager going off at 2:47 a.m. while you are relishing your REM cycle, let me break it down for you. It's like this: a jack hammer angrily drilling into a fleet of fire trucks filled with a legion of the undead.

In fact, it is my belief that if zombies were to harness the power of the pager, they could successfully irritate and exasperate all of humanity into submission, and we would beg them for unfettered relief. It is not enjoyable.

Pages also seem to go off at exactly the most inconvenient time possible.

For example, after you have spent hours preparing a meal that was researched extensively on Pinterest and Food Network.com, and you finally sit down at the table to consume your edible masterpiece.

Typically, that page will come in riiiiighhhhhtttt as you pick up your fork for that very first bite. I don't know about other spouses out there, but I will generally dig right in when this happens. My appetite waits for no one. I do feel a tiny bit guilty about it, though. The good news is, my husband is a record-breaking speed eater. He could be on the phone for a good 15 minutes while I am eating, and still clean his plate before I can even think about what's for dessert.

Pages are also likely to interrupt a hasty shower after a 16-hour day or any sort of bathroom trip. A home catheter would be practical, but just too gross to truly consider.

Memoirs of a Surgeon's Wife, by Megan Sharma

Since each of these interruptions have happened hundreds of times over the better part of a decade, it's only natural that a teeny bit of beeper resentment would begin to well up.

When we lived in Seattle, I dreamed of how I would exact a satisfying revenge on my electronic antagonist:

1. Hop on the Washington State Ferry to Bainbridge Island and slingshot the pager into the Puget Sound, preferably aimed at a loudmouthed seagull for extra points. PETA, if you are reading this, don't you have better things to do? What, are you related to that seagull?

2. Lie in wait in our condo garbage area, hiding in or behind the dumpster, as required. On the pickup day, distract the driver and then slide the pager under the wheel of the gargantuan lime green and orange garbage truck. Listen for a plastic-y crunch. Success!

3. A baseball bat, an empty field. You've seen "Office Space."

4. Drop it from the Space Needle, preferably not onto the neighboring Chihuly Glass Garden. That would be way over budget.

5. Replace any reasonable 30-something person's smart phone with a pager for just one day. That way, you know the deed will be done and you don't have to get your hands dirty.

Memoirs of a Surgeon's Wife, by Megan Sharma

PRIVATE PRACTICE OR ACADEMIC MEDICINE?

Every medical career presents a fork in the road: private practice or academic medicine? True, in the changing face of modern medicine, hybrids do exist (such as working part-time at the Veterans Administration hospital), but these are the most common and traditional routes.

Private practice can take many forms. A physician could inherit or establish his or her own practice, although this trend is on the downward slope for physicians under the age of 40 (Leslie Kane, 2014). Physicians may also choose to join an existing practice. Working for a private, for-profit health care provider or an outpatient clinic can also be considered private practice.

There are other options in between, such as military and government health care.

And then there is the other side of the coin: academic medicine.

Physicians in an academic setting typically work for a university-owned hospital or hospital system. Their work is considered "academic" because it comes with expectations for contributing to the medical and patient community at large through research and leadership activities.

As you might imagine, there are pros and cons to each type of practice.

Some may have dreamt for years of taking over the family practice. For them, it's a foregone conclusion. Others envision total independence over patient care decisions and how to run the business, coupled with nearly unlimited income potential. Being your own boss can sound appealing. Yet, the reality doesn't always match these gleaming images. Insurance and billing hassles, malpractice lawsuits, and the transition to electronic health records can dampen the dream.

Academic physicians are employed—they have a boss and numerous stakeholders to please, in addition to providing excellent patient care. Some physicians in this boat complain of limited decision-making capacity, too many rules and political games, and more limited income potential. Yet, others are happy to avoid shouldering the financial and psychological burden of running their own practice and enjoy a sense of job security, benefits packages for themselves and their families, malpractice protection and a congenial work environment.

There is no right or wrong answer.

If you want to conduct research, work with and teach residents and medical students, share wisdom with your colleagues on the latest in your field, and help educate and empower the broader community, then academic medicine is right up your alley.

If you prefer to focus solely on personal relationships with your patients, clinical practice and/or surgery, then perhaps private practice is a better fit for you.

Who is happier with their career path? It's about even, honestly. Medscape commissioned a 2016 survey of nearly 5,000 U.S. physicians and found that 81 percent of both employed and self-employed physicians feel a great sense of pride and accomplishment in their work (Page, 2016).

Regardless of which fork in the road you choose; I advise you to go with your instincts on people. Your boss and colleagues are people you will see or interact with nearly every day, often in stressful and life-and-death situations. If something feels off or you just don't "click" with the group, give that serious consideration.

For example, when Arun was interviewing for his position as Assistant Professor, he had an uncomfortable experience with a program Department Chair. The Department Chair had made dinner plans with Arun and was to pick him up at his hotel. The Department Chair was nearly an hour late, with no call or text message letting Arun know that he was running late, and no apology upon his eventual arrival. Poor Arun was waiting at the curb of the hotel driveway, growing more and more anxious that he had gotten the time wrong, unsure of what to do.

Memoirs of a Surgeon's Wife, by Megan Sharma

Whereas his current Department Chair is incredibly thoughtful and a wonderful leader. She even made sure to invite me to visit when Arun interviewed and timed it so that I could still travel by plane to join him (I was pregnant at the time). She even arranged for me to have lunch with one of the other doctor's wives while I was in town, in addition to our dinners out and personalized tour of the town.

People demonstrate their best behavior in hiring situations. If they can't even muster a bit of courtesy and decency in early stages, how will they handle things once you've already committed to the job? You may not want to wait to find out.

Memoirs of a Surgeon's Wife, by Megan Sharma

THANKS, BUT NO THANKS

"Want to see what I did at work today?" The answer is no, most certainly not. I *never* want to see what you did at work today, because your job is to cut people open and remove cancer from their body. So…I'm good.

It took me some time to learn this lesson. After seeing dozens of textbook or web images of people with half their faces missing, I caught on.

I mean, I get it. He just wants to show off. It's like when a kid comes home proudly bearing a family portrait they've made at school. Thankfully, I am not obligated to hang my husband's handiwork on the refrigerator. Appetite=gone.

That still doesn't answer the question of why. Why surgical photos and videos? Well, they help others learn. And they are used for research purposes. But mostly to gross out significant others, IMHO.

I will say, however, that I have come to appreciate the surgical videos now that I know more about what's going on. It is some gnarly stuff.

It's like, whoa, the cancer is being blasted away by a laser! Here comes the robot! Except then I see a few drops of blood and I'm like, "Sharma out."

Memoirs of a Surgeon's Wife, by Megan Sharma

WHEN EVERY MEAL IS PROBABLY THE LAST MEAL OF YOUR LIFE

You've heard of athletes carbo-loading before a big competition. Residents feel the need to do this at every opportunity.

Bagels, donuts, and croissants at the weekly conference. Done, done, and done.

It's somebody's birthday? Somebody who works in this hospital but whom I have never met? Woo hoo, let's celebrate by eating a big old slab of chocolate cake! Or two.

Leftover sausage and pepperoni pizza from eight hours ago? Don't mind if I do!

Maybe it's part of the whole starving student mentality. Even though they are already full-blown doctors, technically residents are students. And even more technically they are often broke as hell.

So, every meal is treated like it might be the last.

Another legitimate reason for this phenomenon is long days and sometimes even longer surgeries. Let's just say that residents do not have a designated lunch hour. They are fortunate to get a lunch minute.

Memoirs of a Surgeon's Wife, by Megan Sharma

When food does present itself, eating is anything but graceful. It's all about speed. Shoveling is a preferred method. Chewing is overrated.

When I first met my husband, I was appalled by the lightning speed with which he polished off meals. Although for him, watching me eat slowly was probably akin to watching grass grow. This was a real issue! He would be finished eating before I'd taken my third or fourth bite. It was awkward on dinner dates.

Eventually, after many years, Arun did learn that not every meal was likely to be his last supper. He slowed it on down and stopped eating whatever free junk was lying around.

But this is a tradition that will endure among residents. If the food is free and the empty carbs are plentiful, there they will be.

Memoirs of a Surgeon's Wife, by Megan Sharma

THE VENERABLE ATTENDING: HOW NOT TO ANGER THE GODS

Oh, attendings. They are the bosses. The big kahunas. The kings and queens of the doctors' lounge. The prima donnas of the purgatory that is residency (for their underlings, that is).

How to keep them happy and their wrath at bay?

These are the 10 Commandments for Pleasing Attendings (and bosses everywhere):

1. Thou shalt do what I say and not what I do
2. Thou shalt know when to shut the F up
3. Thou shalt have no other attendings (or priorities) before me
4. Thou shalt not throw me under the bus, even when I am clearly to blame
5. Thou shalt not mock me, lo, though I know not how to type on a computer
6. Thou shalt smile and nod and grit thy teeth
7. Thou shalt read my mind and predict my every whim
8. Thou shalt honor my name and keep it holy
9. Thou shalt remember the Sabbath day and keep on working anyway
10. Thou shalt profusely kiss my ass

Memoirs of a Surgeon's Wife, by Megan Sharma

Follow these commandments and residency will be a cake walk.

Memoirs of a Surgeon's Wife, by Megan Sharma

LET'S REVIEW WHAT KIND OF TALK IS APPROPRIATE AT THE DINNER TABLE

The dinner table. Setting for laughter, sharing a meal, recapping the day that is now in past tense, and making decisions.

Until we bought our new house complete with dining room, ours was a cute little four-person glass table, IKEA 2008. It was nothing special, but it fit perfectly in our open concept living room-kitchen-dining area in Seattle and then in Pittsburgh.

We added pizazz with a set of cherry red dining chairs from Crate and Barrel, each with a price tag exceeding the cost of the original table and its four corresponding POS chairs. Thank you, wedding registry discount! I just couldn't stand fixing the tie-on chair pads (that's right, probably the same ones at your grandmother's house!) for the three thousandth time.

This table was not used exclusively for dining. In fact, it was multi-purpose and accommodated me when I worked from home, became by miniature art studio when I created oil paintings, and was generally a clean surface to throw things on.

From time to time, *some* people in our household seem to develop a keen lack of social understanding of what kind of talk is appropriate at the dinner table.

Memoirs of a Surgeon's Wife, by Megan Sharma

Examples of things I prefer not to hear about during the evening meal:
- Bodily expulsions or leakages
- Reasons for changing scrubs mid-day
- Squirting, pumping, or spraying blood patterns
- Things that can be accomplished with a hand saw
- Interesting uses for redundant thigh tissue

While I recognize that these are equivalent to my thrilling tales of mind-numbing meetings and variations on the standard nonfat cappuccino, I just can't stomach the surgeon's "shop talk" while eating.

Memoirs of a Surgeon's Wife, by Megan Sharma

BOOT CAMP OR RESIDENCY?

I have never served in the U.S. armed forces. Shoot, I've never even held a gun (pun intended!). So, my perceptions of military basic training (boot camp) are primarily culled from the stories my grandfathers have told, TV, movies, and the research I've done for this book. I cannot help but recognize similarities between boot camp and medical residency. There's nothing like a good old side-by-side comparison, so, here goes.

Boot Camp	Residency
Required for all American service members	Required for all American medical school graduates
"Transforms civilians into soldiers" (U.S. Army)	"Your residency is important because it's a time of tremendous growth both in your clinical knowledge base as well as your professional development. Much of what you learn will come from patients." (Association of American Medical Colleges)
"Over the course of ten weeks, recruits will learn basic tactical and survival skills along with how to shoot, rappel, and march. They will also learn the basics of Army life and military customs, including the Seven Core Army Values." (U.S. Army)	Residents learn survival skills, minus the rappelling and marching part.
Seven to 12-week training	Three to eight-year residency

Memoirs of a Surgeon's Wife, by Megan Sharma

program, depending on the military branch	program, depending on specialty
Recruits won't earn the full respect of their leaders and peers until graduation day, or even beyond	Residents won't earn the full respect of their leaders and peers until graduation day, or at least until they become senior or chief residents, and sometimes not even until they become senior attending physicians
"The supreme quality for leadership is unquestionably integrity. Without it, no real success is possible, no matter whether it is on a section gang, a football field, in an army, or in an office." –General Dwight D. Eisenhower	"He who studies medicine without books sails an uncharted sea, but he who studies medicine without patients does not go to sea at all." – William Osler
An incredible test of character and strength	An incredible test of character and strength
Not self, but country (U.S. Navy)	First, do no harm (Hippocrates)

Like peanut butter and jelly. Who knew?

I would also like to give a heartfelt shout-out to all the military members and families out there. Thank you for your service to our country. Your strength inspires me!

"From this day to the ending of the world,
But we in it shall be remembered-
We few, we happy few, we band of brothers;
For he to-day that sheds his blood with me
Shall be my brother; be he ne'er so vile,
This day shall gentle his condition;
And gentlemen in England now-a-bed
Shall think themselves accurs'd they were not here,
And hold their manhoods cheap whiles any speaks
That fought with us upon Saint Crispin's day."
— William Shakespeare in his most famous "war play," "Henry V"

Memoirs of a Surgeon's Wife, by Megan Sharma

ALL IN A DAY'S WORK

Okay, so working in a hospital or doctor's office isn't exactly akin to the inherent danger of operating a nuclear power plant. It does come with certain on-the-job hazards and other inconveniences, however.

We'll start with hazards. Needle sticks and blood spatters (to the eyes, nose, mouth or broken skin) are common and require immediate testing for Hepatitis B/C and HIV. This happened to Arun a few times during residency, and it is alarming, especially when working with high-risk patients at the county hospital (homeless folks, drug addicts, prostitutes, prisoners, etc.). My stomach always tightened when Arun told me that he had sustained a needle stick or a cut from a surgical instrument, even though the test results always came back negative.

Working in a county hospital also means annual Tuberculosis (TB) vaccinations and testing. A shot is a shot, but the tuberculin skin test is rather unpleasant. Per WebMD, the test is done by putting a small amount of TB protein (antigens) under the top layer of skin on the inner forearm. If the person has ever been exposed to the TB bacteria (Mycobacterium tuberculosis), their skin will react to the antigens by developing a firm red bump at the site within two days (WebMD, 2016).

Tuberculosis was virtually wiped out in the 1950s with the help of antibiotics, but the disease has resurfaced recently in potent, drug-resistant forms. Since TB sufferers typically don't demonstrate any symptoms and the disease can be latent or active, testing for health care workers is critical (WebMD, 2016).

Now, for an inconvenience. And who does inconvenience and bureaucracy better than government agencies? The VA requires residents to be fingerprinted every four years. Since Arun had a six-year residency, he had to go through this process twice—visiting the police station and all.

Will someone please explain to me the point of this whole exercise? Do fingerprints change? Does the VA suspect that residents are secretly shaving down their finger pads in their plentiful free time? Ah, the mysteries of the universe.

It's all in a day's work.

Memoirs of a Surgeon's Wife, by Megan Sharma

A WORD TO MOTHERS WHO ASPIRE TO HAVE A SURGEON-IN-LAW

Oh, you moms out there (I now count myself a member of your prestigious ranks, so I can say that). You want the very best for your children. And I mean the *very* best. We're talking champagne wishes and caviar dreams, ya'll. And who could blame us?

Maybe you, like my amazing in-laws, decided to leave everything behind in your early thirties so that your five-year-old son and future children would have a better life in a country thousands of miles from where your ancestors were born.

Perhaps you quit a lucrative corporate job to stay home with your sweet baby girl.

Or maybe you saved your pennies to send each of your kids to college debt-free. That is a special gift.

Simply put, we want it all for our offspring. And we want them to find the right person to share their lives with.

We pray that our daughters will meet and marry a man who is loving, kind, patient, funny, good looking, and smart. Not "The Bachelor." Oh, god, no. Someone who has his shit together.

Memoirs of a Surgeon's Wife, by Megan Sharma

If you think "Dr. Prince Charming" has a nice ring to it, you're probably not alone. Just think of all the free medical advice! *How should I treat a migraine? Do I need to take supplements? What shall I do about these warts?* Such great fun!

I'm here to offer a bit of a reality check to mothers who aspire to have a surgeon-in-law (SIL):

- If you imagined getting out of those regular mammograms and colonoscopies, think again. Your SIL is going to make sure you get those done, come hell or high water.
- You're going to have the safest grandbabies ever! But you will often find yourself saying, "Well, my kids did it, and they survived!"
- You will get free medical advice, but it will sometimes irritate your darling SIL (especially if you constantly ask questions outside of his or her area of expertise).
- More than likely, your son or daughter and his/her family will be moving to advance your SIL's career. Possibly more than once, and possibly for good.
- Your SIL will likely know more about your health status than you will. SILs can read between the lines.

My mom loves her SIL dearly and I'm sure she would carry the banner for other moms out there who want to join the club.

The club is cool. The club comes with a free lifetime subscription to Health and Family Circle. Just kidding.

Memoirs of a Surgeon's Wife, by Megan Sharma

SEEKING YOUR ADVICE

Subject: Your expertise and advice: URGENT!!!!

Dear Arun,

I hope you and your family are doing well. I'm writing to seek your wisdom and advice. A very close family member is in need.

My wife's sister's cousin's sister (didi) in Delhi has recently been experiencing problems swallowing. She visited a well-acclaimed ENT in Delhi, who examined her throat and ran some tests. The doctor recommended further treatment. I have attached a copy of her scans.

However, before we move forward with more medical interventions, we would be most grateful for your expertise on this matter. Please do call us to discuss.

Many, many blessings to you and we eagerly anticipate speaking with you.

Warmest wishes,

Distant family friend of your parents in India (whom you have never met)

Memoirs of a Surgeon's Wife, by Megan Sharma

WHY EVERYONE SHOULD HAVE A RESEARCH YEAR (BUT NOT MORE THAN ONE)

I am so thankful for that full year of research time my husband had during his residency. Not every residency program has that kind of protected research time, but the University of Washington does.

For Arun, I know it was strange to suddenly become an office dweller for the first time ever. Being a desk potato and being a scalpel jockey are two very different positions. It was especially hard for him not to be able to do surgery since he didn't have hospital privileges during this time.

Plus, he had to dress up for work every day. No more defaulting to scrubs if he slept in too late.

There were a few things I loved about this time. Primarily, this was when we did the heavy lifting of our wedding planning. It was like a wedding planning boot camp and we got through it together and efficiently. Our favorite part was the food tasting. Arun wouldn't have been available to meet with vendors or participate much in the planning if he were in his typically insane residency routine.

We were also able to carpool to work together, a first for us. Having more consistent office hours also meant that we could eat dinner together. Mind blown!

Memoirs of a Surgeon's Wife, by Megan Sharma

Most importantly, the research year gave Arun the opportunity to feel like a normal human being again and to catch up on sleep, if only for a little while. He could see friends, watch TV, visit the gym, and set the alarm clock later than 4:00 a.m.

But a year away from the hospital nearly bored my dear husband to death. Don't get me wrong, he truly enjoys research and it's a big part of his practice today, but he is better on his feet and taking care of patients than answering endless emails.

Therefore, given the option, one year of research is better than two.

Memoirs of a Surgeon's Wife, by Megan Sharma

PLEDGING THE FRATERNITY, I MEAN, FITTING IN

It's no state secret that the world of medicine, and surgery in particular, have long been a boys' club.

There is no official history of American women in medicine until the mid-1800s, even though medicine has been a part of our nation since colonial times, with doctors grappling with little-understood disease and widespread infant mortality (Wikipedia, 2016).

In the Victorian era, it was generally believed that no respectable woman would have interest in a career in medicine. Think about it: getting up close and personal with the human body (nudity!), treating debilitating and deadly diseases, and plenty of blood and gore. This is the life of a physician, and it is certainly not suited for a "proper" lady, or so it was thought.

Yet, there was one such woman by the name of Elizabeth Blackwell who had concluded that her teaching career was neither intellectually stimulating nor fulfilling. When a dying friend confided in Elizabeth that her suffering could have been lessened had she been attended by a woman physician, Elizabeth decided to pursue the medical profession (U.S. National Library of Medicine, 2016).

In 1849 Dr. Elizabeth Blackwell was the first woman to receive an M.D. degree from an American medical school, graduating first in her class, no less (National Library of Medicine, 2016). That doesn't mean it was easy for her.

Memoirs of a Surgeon's Wife, by Megan Sharma

Dr. Joseph Warrington, a well-respected physician who eventually became a friend, advised Elizabeth, who had received rejection after rejection from U.S. medical schools: "Elizabeth, it is of no use trying. Thee cannot gain admission to these schools. Thee must go to Paris and don masculine attire to gain the necessary knowledge." (U.S. National Library of Medicine, 2016)

Elizabeth didn't throw in the towel, and she certainly didn't disguise herself as a man to gain entry. She pressed on.

"She convinced two physician friends to let her read medicine with them for a year and applied to all the medical schools in New York and Philadelphia. She also applied to twelve more schools in the northeast states and was accepted by Geneva Medical College in western New York state in 1847. The faculty, assuming that the all-male student body would never agree to a woman joining their ranks, allowed them to vote on her admission. As a joke, they voted yes, and she gained admittance, despite the reluctance of most students and faculty." (National Library of Medicine, 2016)

In medical school Elizabeth faced outright disdain and ridicule from her male peers, who simply could not understand her shared presence. Even her professors presented obstacles, including a reluctance to allow her to participate in lectures on reproductive anatomy. Elizabeth insisted on being treated the same as every other student. She continued to exhibit a focus and determination to excel in her studies (U.S. National Library of Medicine, 2016).

By graduation day, she had won the respect and admiration of the students, faculty and townspeople of Geneva.

The Dean of the college, Dr. Charles A. Lee, delivered a graduation address in January 1849 that expressly recognized Elizabeth's hard-earned achievement:

> An event connected with the proceedings of this day deserves some notice on this occasion, calculated as it is to excite curiosity and comment, and to be held up as an example for other institutions to imitate or condemn. I mean the conferring of the degree of M.D. upon one of that sex which is generally supposed to be wanting in the physical, if not moral qualifications necessary for the successful practice of the Healing Art. So far as I am informed, this is the first instance, in this country, or any other, where a female has graduated in medicine, after having gone through the

Memoirs of a Surgeon's Wife, by Megan Sharma

regular prescribed course and term of study...This, I say, deserves as it will receive, the heart-felt approbation of every generous and humane mind. This event will stand forth hereafter as a memorable example of what woman can undertake and accomplish, too, when stimulated by the love of science and a noble spirit of philanthropy. (Charles A. Lee, 1849)

Dr. Lee then goes on to make some remarks that previous generations of physicians could never have imagined being uttered. He says, "Why should medical science be monopolized by us alone? Why should woman be prohibited from fulfilling her mission as a ministering angel to the sick, furnished not only with the softer and kindlier attributes of her sex, but with all the appliances and resources of science? If she feels called to this life of toil and responsibility, and gives evidence of her qualifications for such a calling, in humanity's name, let her take her rank among the disciples of Aesculapius, and be honored for her self-sacrificing choice." (Charles A. Lee, 1849)

Then Dr. Lee turns right around, in his very next sentence, and pulls a serious dick move. "Such cases must be *ever too few*, to disturb the existing relations of society, or excite any other feeling on our part than admiration at the heroism displayed, and sympathy, for the sufferings voluntarily assumed!" (Charles A. Lee, 1849)

So, this is cool and unique and all, guys—but let's not let it happen again. It would make all of us men feel uncomfortable and it might even jeopardize our standing as the supreme rulers of the universe. Just say no to ladies in medicine.

Dr. Lee even went so far as to include a lengthy footnote in the printed version of his valedictory address making his position on women in medicine perfectly clear.

> The writer [Dr. Lee], while he acknowledges the validity of the argument, so far as it is founded on the general physical disqualifications of the sex for the medical profession, and the incompatibility of its duties, with those properly belonging to the female portion of society, believes, nevertheless, that instances occasionally happen, where females display such a combination of moral, physical, and intellectual qualifications for discharging creditably and skillfully the duties belonging to our calling, that it would seem equally unwise and unjust, to withhold from them those advantages and those honors, which are open to nearly all others, whether deserving of them or not. (Charles A. Lee, 1849)

Memoirs of a Surgeon's Wife, by Megan Sharma

Dr. Lee also "feels bound to say, that the inconveniences attending the admission of females to all the lectures in a medical school are so great, that he will feel compelled on all future occasions, to oppose such a practice..." (Charles A. Lee, 1849).

Medical school graduation, however, was just the beginning for this incredible young woman.

Dr. Blackwell championed the medical careers of numerous women when she founded the New York Infirmary for Women and Children in 1857, a full-scale hospital serving both medical and surgical patients. By establishing this institution, Dr. Blackwell not only served the poor, she also "offered a practical solution to one of the problems facing women who were rejected from internships elsewhere but determined to expand their skills as physicians" (National Library of Medicine, 2016). This institution still exists as the New York University Downtown Hospital.

She fought for women's rights throughout her life and published several important books on the issue of women in medicine, including "Medicine: A Profession For Women" in 1860 and "Address on the Medical Education of Women" in 1864 (National Library of Medicine, 2016).

When Dr. Blackwell realized that women were still being denied admittance to the all-male medical colleges of the time, she knew what she had to do: establish her own women's medical college. The Woman's Medical College of New York Infirmary opened in 1868, with 15 students and a faculty of nine, including Elizabeth and her younger sister, Emily (National Library of Medicine, 2016).

In 1869 Dr. Blackwell returned to the country of her birth, England, to continue her career lecturing and running her own private practice. She left the medical college in New York under the directorship of her sister. Dr. Blackwell spent the remaining 40 years of her life in Great Britain, after contributing so much to her adopted country, America (National Library of Medicine, 2016).

Medicine has come a long way toward gender inclusivity since 1849. But even more than 165 years later, as one might expect, we're not "there" yet.

As of 2014, nearly 50 percent of American medical students and residents were women (AAMC, 2016). Yet in the same year, only 38 percent of full time faculty and 21 percent of full professors were women (AAMC, 2016).

Memoirs of a Surgeon's Wife, by Megan Sharma

It gets even more interesting when you examine the distribution of male and female residents by specialty. As of 2013, the specialties with the highest overall percentages of women residents were, perhaps not surprisingly, Obstetrics and Gynecology (82.6 percent women), Pediatrics (70.6 percent women), and Allergy and Immunology (65.9 percent women) (AAMC, 2016).

On the other hand, the specialties with the lowest overall percentages of women residents in 2013 were Orthopedic Surgery (13.8 percent women), Neurological Surgery (15.8 percent women), and Thoracic Surgery (19.8 percent women) (AAMC, 2016).

For my husband's specialty, Otolaryngology, in 2013 there were 522 women residents and 1,505 men residents—that's 34.7 percent women (AAMC, 2016).

Of all residents across specialties in 2013, only 45.9 percent were women. This number only rose slightly from 40.7 percent in 2003, 10 years prior (AAMC, 2016).

From this data, one could conclude that even in recent years, women are still the minority in the residency programs that are so critical on the career path of a physician. Putting these women at an even greater disadvantage, female leadership lags further behind.

In the field of Otolaryngology, as you move up the faculty ranks from Instructor to Assistant Professor to Associate Professor to Full Professor, the number of women plummets. In 2014 only 9 percent of Full Professors in Otolaryngology were women—this represents 32 women nationwide (AAMC, 2016). That is the third lowest percentage across the board, with only Orthopedic Surgery (five percent women) and Surgery (eight percent women) demonstrating lower percentages of Full Professors being women.

In the Clinical Sciences (from Internal Medicine to Anesthesiology to General Surgery and everything in between), only 19 percent of Full Professors are women. Thirty-six percent of all Faculty, across ranks, are women (AAMC, 2016). There simply are not enough women faculty to look up to and to learn from.

And what about women in leadership positions to mentor, support, and stand up for their female colleagues? Very tough to find.

Memoirs of a Surgeon's Wife, by Megan Sharma

At the institution where my husband completed his residency program, as of December 2013, in Otolaryngology, there were 16 men and only one woman Department Chair (AAMC, 2016).

This is a challenging reality. It is simply easier for male residents to connect with male colleagues and leaders than for female residents to do the same. Given the high-pressure work environment, the age gaps and the competitive drive to succeed, it can become awkward for both trainees and faculty to have meaningful professional relationships with the opposite sex. Furthermore, it is difficult, if not impossible, for male mentors to advise female mentees on balancing family and career, or how to handle the time off required to start a family.

When women do make their way to the top, they are still paid less than their male counterparts. A study published in September 2016 by The Journal of the American Medical Association (JAMA) Network revealed stunning sex differences in physician salaries in U.S. public medical schools. Among more than 10,000 physicians analyzed, female physicians earned, on average, nearly $20,000 less than male physicians, even after adjusting the analysis for age, experience, specialty, faculty rank, research productivity, and clinical revenue. Furthermore, female full professors earned salaries comparable to those of male associate professors, a lower rank. (Anupam B. Jena, Olenski, & Daniel M. Blumenthal, 2016).

We can only speculate about the great divide in pay equity in private practice settings, which, unlike many public institutions, are not required to publish employee salary information.

How does this imbalance of power manifest itself in the workplace?

Surgical residency is very much like pledging a fraternity. There is history. There is culture. There are spoken and unspoken rules of conduct. There are founding members and luminaries to be admired. Loyalty and trust are critical. It is a male-dominated field. There is a leading train of thought that whatever one person endured as a resident, others who follow must also endure. And then there are the pranks.

I talked with one of my female surgeon friends, who described a few such pranks she witnessed during her residency (just a few years ago).

One involved filling a male resident's white coat pockets with lubricant. Another prank was a phone mouth and ear piece covered in lube. How original.

Memoirs of a Surgeon's Wife, by Megan Sharma

According to my friend, acting like "one of the boys" was part of the job. And none of these pranks were ever pulled on a female resident.

And then, of course, there were the off-color jokes and comments permeating the (professional?!?) working environment. Inappropriate references to laryngoscopy (things going down the throat), bending over, and detailed recounts of the physical appearance of female colleagues, to name a few examples.

The grossest illustration of male chauvinism was this: a male attending (an authority figure) who would wear his pager centered right over his crotch during surgery, so that the nurses would have to grab it in that uncomfortable location to answer his pages. Ugh.

Is it any wonder that many female physicians feel like they are in an uphill battle to fit in?

Since you have gotten this far into the chapter, it probably won't surprise you to learn that hazing still exists in medical training.

This is a story imparted by another surgeon friend who recently became an attending physician.

One of my most unforgettable moments during my intern year was on a surgery sub-specialty rotation (not my own sub-specialty). I watched all week as the senior residents ragged on a junior resident. They were relentless in their verbal abuse of him—his physical appearance, personality, patient care, surgical work, everything.

Once that same junior resident got bodily fluids on his scrubs, as tends to happen in our line of work. His seniors told him that he was disgusting. Rather than giving him the opportunity to change clothes, I watched as one senior resident held him down and sprayed a sticky skin pre-treatment (used to help make tape stick) down his pants and then cut off the offending soiled pant leg with trauma shears.

When the junior resident went into the bathroom to change and then realized he grabbed the wrong pants size, he asked the senior residents to give him the correct size. His seniors "kindly" gave him a new pair of scrub bottoms, as requested. However, they gave him pants sized far too small.

Memoirs of a Surgeon's Wife, by Megan Sharma

That was the breaking point for him that day. He threw an all-out fit in the bathroom: screaming, hitting, and throwing things. It lasted at least 20 minutes and the whole time his senior residents were talking about how he had it so good and shouldn't complain. They'd had it much worse when they were junior residents.

True, it's not like this everywhere. There are plenty of institutions which value the contributions of men and women equally. And I would venture to say that most male doctors and surgeons of my generation have a huge amount of respect for their female colleagues.

But should it be like this *anywhere*? That's where the real dialogue should begin.

Memoirs of a Surgeon's Wife, by Megan Sharma

IF YOU DO NOT PUT THAT PHONE DOWN I AM GOING TO THROW IT IN THE TOILET

I have a thing. A thing about phones. Here it is: there are certain times and places where phones do not belong.

I am certainly not the first to ban the presence of a smart phone at the dinner table, and I won't be the last. It's particularly egregious when you are married to a doctor because you feel like that phone *owns* you both. Texting, calling, email—it never stops. Patient care never stops.

But I must give Arun credit. I think I only threatened to throw his phone in the toilet once or twice before he understood how I treasure and need just one uninterrupted conversation per day. His full attention. Time is love, right?

Now, as parents, we both need to be careful. We keep that little rectangular screen away from our daughter at all costs. We don't want her to think that we love our Facebook alerts more than we love her little toothy smile. No contest.

Our relationships are better off. And so is our plumbing.

Memoirs of a Surgeon's Wife, by Megan Sharma

GUESS WHAT'S IN MY WORK BAG?

What a person carries with them to work says a lot about them.

What do you think a surgeon would carry? Allow me to dispel any wild rumors on this topic. Here is an inventory of Arun's work messenger bag on an average, fairly cleaned out day of residency:

- Four pairs of clean scrubs
- A thick wad of papers
- One head lamp
- Mini deodorant
- Two toothbrushes
- Eye drops
- Two surgical marking pens (purple, my favorite color)
- Lunch leftovers from three weeks ago, including one appetizing plastic baggie of emulsified carrot
- Not one, but two pairs of spare glasses that are likely several years behind on the prescription
- One tongue depressor
- One absorbable suture pack
- One excessively heavy laptop
- *Notably missing: any semblance of a life outside hospital doors*

Memoirs of a Surgeon's Wife, by Megan Sharma

DON'T BE SUCH A DUMMY

Here is some free medical advice from me, an untrained non-medical professional who clearly still knows everything about everything. Take it for what it's worth (<a grain of salt).

If something is growing on your body that doesn't belong there...go, see the doctor!

If part of your face is eroding away...go, see the doctor!

If you're living with chronic, undiagnosed pain...go, see the doctor!

If you gain or lose weight faster than "The Biggest Loser"...go, see the doctor!

If you constantly smell like mothballs and expired gorgonzola...go, see the doctor!

If you have been putting off that doctor's appointment for seven years...go, see the doctor!

If you smoke and drink like there's no tomorrow and can no longer swallow...go, see the doctor!

If you think you don't need no damn medicine...go, see the doctor!

Memoirs of a Surgeon's Wife, by Megan Sharma

Don't be such a dummy, dummy...go, see the doctor!

Memoirs of a Surgeon's Wife, by Megan Sharma

FOR THE LOVE OF DANSKOS

I totally get the concept of work shoes. Sturdy boots for firemen and construction workers, seven-inch clear plastic heels for strippers, and polished oxfords or Cole Haan pumps for the business world.

In the medical community, it's all about the Danskos.

Danskos are perhaps the ugliest shoes to grace God's green earth. They look like knockoff Dutch clogs and are worn as slip on shoes.

To add insult to injury, these suckers are expensive. The basic styles start around $120.00, up to $150.00. Granted, they do wear well and only need replacing every four years or so. I guess that's a plus.

Danskos come in a variety of colors and styles, from patent leather to pebble leather to extra, extra shiny patent leather. Flowers, stripes, psychedelic swirls, sequins, spots, you name it. I guess that makes them "stylish," or something. I'm sticking with something.

I wish I could tell you exactly how many medical professionals (medical assistants/nurses/physician assistants/primary care docs/surgeons/anesthesiologists/radiologists) wear Danskos, but I couldn't find any concrete data. My guess is 70 percent.

When asked why he wears them, my husband said, "Because it's easy to clean blood from them."

Memoirs of a Surgeon's Wife, by Megan Sharma

    Well, there you have it. The bloodless wonder shoes. They practically sell themselves.

Memoirs of a Surgeon's Wife, by Megan Sharma

BAD ASS WOMEN IN MEDICINE

Female physicians have to fight every day—for acknowledgment, for respect, for chances.

Dr. Allyson Herbst, an internal medicine resident at Emory University, described some of her experiences and struggles in an October 2016 article for "The Washington Post." As a medical student in New York, Dr. Herbst recalled a conversation with a resident physician that made her stomach turn. As they weighed various specialty options over lunch, including internal medicine and obstetrics/gynecology, he asked (with obvious pleasure), "Do you like vagina?" Later that week, the same male resident chastised Dr. Herbst for not wearing makeup, saying, "You're not wearing make-up today. Maybe you should rethink that choice." (Herbst, 2016)

In the few short days following publication of Dr. Herbst's article, more than 600 comments were posted online. One commentator noted that part way through his/her mother's interview for medical school, the interviewer leaned back and asked, "So, why does a blonde want to be a physician?"

Another commentator said, "As a physician I can attest that what she says is true. Unfortunately, there is a pervading culture, mainly in surgical specialties, to treat women like objects. I have been very outspoken on this issue and sometimes I have displeased my male colleagues, but this behavior is common and in certain places the worst offenders are the ones in charge."

Memoirs of a Surgeon's Wife, by Megan Sharma

Other more aggressive (mostly male) commentators accused Dr. Herbst of "whining" and overstating the issue. One woman even said, "Lady, stop whining and go to work."

After reading through dozens of hateful, sexist and ignorant comments from men and women alike, I couldn't take it anymore. I closed the article. Can you imagine being the woman these comments are directed toward?

Why do these brave women do it? How do they persevere through the flying garbage? I wanted to know what makes them tick.

Three amazing surgeon friends who happen to be women were kind enough to indulge me and share their thoughts and experiences.

The first is "Sophia" (name has been changed). Sophia's parents pushed her and her older brother toward medicine. There was a huge amount of cultural pressure to go down that road. Sophia focused heavily on math and science in high school and volunteered at a hospital, but she hardly imagined that one day she would be taking people apart and then putting them back together again.

In medical school, a mentor of Sophia's who was also a woman told her that she was "too nice" to be a surgeon. This hit Sophia particularly hard, especially because she had known the woman for several years and felt confident in her own abilities. But Sophia didn't give up her dream of becoming a surgeon. She kept on moving toward her goal.

There were other obstacles. Sophia did not immediately place into the residency program she was aiming for. She had to wait a year and strategize to find the best path to her desired specialty. When she did match to a program the following year, she was overjoyed. She never even interviewed in person and still got the job. That was one of her proudest moments, she said.

Once in her residency, Sophia learned that some things are easier when you're a girl, like getting the early bird special at Jiffy Lube an hour late, or foul-mouthed attendings toning it down in her presence, but other things are more difficult. "Too friendly" male attendings and no one to go to, for starters. More scrutiny and quick judgment on mistakes, as well. But the biggest challenge, she said, was the lack of a female support system in the workplace.

Memoirs of a Surgeon's Wife, by Megan Sharma

Sophia noted an interesting difference in how she was treated by the women around her. Female nurses and patients gave her more attitude, were snippier, and often demonstrated a lack of trust in her. Whereas her male colleagues were automatically given deference, because men are expected to be doctors. There were many times she was confused for a nurse. And as a young-looking woman, at times her patients were concerned about the care they would receive, based on her appearance alone.

There were scary and intense moments. Like the time she had a patient who was in a devastating car wreck, blood pulsing from his/her face and flailing all over the place while Sophia struggled to secure an airway. Amid the chaos, Sophia stuck her finger into the patient's neck to secure the tracheotomy, saving his/her life.

Sophia says that you learn things as a medical student that just don't prepare you for the reality of medicine under pressure. She also never expected to treat patients who have suffered a bear attack, but she has done it, and she loves the adrenaline rush of her job.

Her advice to aspiring surgeons is: "You can do it! But you have to love what you do." She also wants you to know that "Grey's Anatomy" is entertaining but not very realistic.

Next, we have "Chloe" (name has been changed). This is how Chloe describes herself: "I am, admittedly, a very direct type A personality. I deal with problems directly and am almost never passive-aggressive. When I am at work, I focus on work and social time comes later. I was raised to be self-sufficient, confident (or to at least project it even when I am not), and independent. I was a competitive college athlete. I can change my own oil. I don't need anyone to lift anything for me. I am not easily intimidated. I am not unfriendly, but I do not fit the expectations of a typically more friendly, social, deferring woman."

Characteristics very much in line with a successful career, and not at all uncommon in the surgical field.

Yet, Chloe often dealt with feedback that she was too harsh. She was once called into the nursing manager's office for "intimidating the nurses" because she had chosen to discuss patient care issues directly with those nurses, rather than to do it in a roundabout way.

Memoirs of a Surgeon's Wife, by Megan Sharma

Chloe's evaluations during her first two years of residency training frequently mentioned that she did a good job and patients liked her, but she was too direct, too assertive, and not friendly enough. When Chloe asked for examples, she was told that she didn't smile or chat with the staff enough and was too focused on getting the job done. Hence, she received these unofficial labels: bitchy, difficult, and unfriendly.

Fast forward four years, and many of those same staff members and attending physicians had finally gotten used to Chloe's way of doing things—she still keeps in touch with many of them.

Chloe remembers with great clarity these in-person evaluations:

Male attending physician (who just finished telling Chloe he thinks she really improved on the service): "You know senior resident X is a really good role model for you. She is outgoing and friendly. She often wears makeup. Have you thought about wearing makeup? Maybe some lipstick?"

Female attending physician: "I appreciate that you show up in clinic clothes. We sometimes have a hard time getting the residents to dress for clinic. However, I think you are sometimes over-dressing. You should make sure that you don't look nicer than the attending."

Chloe's written evaluation from the same female attending: "Dr. X is well-prepared in clinic. She arrives on time and is consistently appropriately dressed in clinic clothes, which is a refreshing change from her peers, who arrive in scrubs."

And then there is "Amelia" (name has been changed). Amelia says it's insane what some people can live through. She once had a patient who was water tubing from the back of a jet ski. After the rope became wrapped around his/her neck and he/she was pulled underwater and even had a stroke, he/she left the hospital walking and talking and, most importantly, alive.

Amelia says the best part of her job is operating and solving problems. She is less enthused about getting too involved in social work, trying to please attendings, and general BS. Having gotten this far already helps motivate her to keep going.

She has noticed that some of the attendings are easier on women. It's nice to avoid getting yelled at, but does this mean that they have lower expectations, she

Memoirs of a Surgeon's Wife, by Megan Sharma

wonders? Now, with a few years of residency under her belt, Amelia feels more certain that male residents are held to a higher standard and generally pushed harder than their female counterparts.

Amelia admits that part of it may be "our problem" as women—in that women are more inclined to hand over surgical instruments when told to do so, whereas men will hold on and keep going.

When Amelia considers her future after residency, she worries about succeeding in an academic setting while balancing her personal life. "How will I ever be productive enough to get promoted with all the other responsibilities at home?" And, the alternative? "You'll be having kids at 45," she says.

Amelia concurs with Sophia on the observation that with female colleagues there are often more opportunities for second guessing and disrespect. She is pleased to report that this phenomenon tends to improve over time.

She, too, has had frightening moments. There was one instance with a thyroid cancer patient who had a very narrow and difficult airway and a high risk of bleeding out. She had to secure the patient's trach (airway) early in the morning when no one else was around (as a junior resident, a newbie)—helping the patient breathe manually with a bag in the process. There were a terrifying 30 seconds when she thought her patient was going to die. Despite the blood and pus spewing everywhere, Amelia put the trach back in and the patient survived.

Amelia advises future surgeons to take everything day to day. There are good days and bad days, she says.

The difference is this: when you're a doctor, on the bad days, people may die. When you're an office worker, a bad day is when your boss sends you an irritating email or you get stuck with a project you don't want to deal with. It's all about perspective.

Speaking of perspective, let's briefly consider what it has been like for women in the United States since Dr. Elizabeth Blackwell paved the way by earning her medical degree in 1849.

In 1860, Dr. Blackwell described the stronghold of societal pressure for women to conform to certain approved vocational endeavors. "The interests and occupations of women, as they actually are at present, may be referred to four

Memoirs of a Surgeon's Wife, by Megan Sharma

distinct forms of effort: Domestic life; the education of youth; social intercourse; and benevolent effort of various kinds... Social intercourse—a very limited thing in a half civilized country, becomes in our centres of civilization a great power, establishing customs more binding than laws, imposing habits and stamping opinions, a tribunal from whose judgment there is hardly an appeal." (Dr. Elizabeth Blackwell, 1860)

And then Dr. Blackwell puts the need for women in the profession of medicine in the simplest of terms that surely everyone can understand. "The medical profession is at present too far removed from the life of women; they regard these subjects from such a different stand-point that they can not supply the want. The application of scientific knowledge to women's necessities in actual life can only be done by women who possess the scientific learning of the physician, and as women a thorough acquaintance with women's requirements—that is, by women physicians." (Dr. Elizabeth Blackwell, 1860)

Care for women by women. It doesn't sound revolutionary, but in fact, it was. Men had always dominated the field of medicine.

Other brave women followed suit. Dr. Rebecca Crumpler became the first African American woman in the United States to receive a medical degree in 1864. Following the end of the Civil War, Dr. Crumpler joined other African American physicians caring for freed slaves who would otherwise have no access to medical care. In 1883 Dr. Crumpler published her "Book of Medical Discourses", an exceptionally rare accomplishment for an African American in her day and age (U.S. National Library of Medicine, 2016).

Although she was not a physician, Clara Barton put herself directly in the line of danger during the Civil War to comfort, nurse, and cook for the wounded. She founded the American Red Cross in 1881 (American Red Cross, 2016).

In the many decades leading into the 20th century and beyond, other American women made their mark in medicine.

Dr. Bertha Van Hoosen, who went on to establish the American Medical Women's Association in 1915, encountered many obstacles over the course of her career. Bertha's parents refused to finance her education, and yet she earned both her bachelor's degree and her medical degree. After gaining experience via private practice, Dr. Van Hoosen was made a professor of gynecology at the Illinois University Medical School, even though her appointment was opposed by the all-

Memoirs of a Surgeon's Wife, by Megan Sharma

male faculty. As an outspoken champion of women's rights, Dr. Van Hoosen grew increasingly vocal regarding the medical establishment's discriminatory treatment of women. After being barred from the Chicago Gynecological and Obstetrical Society and feeling isolated within the American Medical Association, she gathered a meeting of women in Chicago that eventually led to the formation of the American Medical Women's Association (American Medical Women's Association, 2016). It was not until 1997 that Dr. Nancy Dickey was elected as the first female president of the American Medical Association (American Medical Association, 2016).

Women don't always receive the accolades and credit they deserve. A prime example of this is the brilliant chemist Rosalind Franklin, whose studies of x-ray diffraction provided critical clues to the structure of DNA. While Rosalind died young after suffering from ovarian cancer, her colleagues James Watson, Francis Crick, and Maurice Wilkins were awarded the Nobel Prize for discovering the shape of our genetic makeup—the double helix—after viewing x-ray photographs of DNA taken by Rosalind. She was not recognized for her contribution until long after her death (U.S. National Library of Medicine, 2016).

Another example is Dr. Mary Edwards Walker, who was the first woman awarded the Congressional Medal of Honor for her work as a surgeon during the Civil War. Her name was removed from the list of honorees in 1917, along with others, during a period of turmoil over award eligibility. According to her biography by the U.S. National Library of Medicine, Dr. Walker remained proud of her achievement and "refused to surrender the medal...and continued to wear it for the rest of her life." Many years after her death, thanks to efforts of her family and a reappraisal of her work by Congress, the honor was finally restored to Dr. Walker in 1977 (U.S. National Library of Medicine, 2016).

There are numerous inspiring women in medicine. In fact—too many to mention here. Especially noteworthy are Dr. Virginia Apgar and her first standardized test to evaluate infants; Dr. Mary Dixon Jones, a world-renowned surgeon credited as the first person in the U.S. to propose and perform a full hysterectomy; and Dr. Gerty Cori, the first woman in America to receive a Nobel Prize in science (along with her husband, Dr. Carl Cori) (U.S. National Library of Medicine, 2016).

And then there are women from others parts of the world like Madame Marie Curie, winner of two Nobel Prizes for her work in radioactivity, who was no stranger to heartache and struggle. After sharing her first Nobel Prize in the field of nuclear physics with her husband, Pierre Curie, and colleague, Henry Becquerel, in

1903, she suffered a tragic loss. Pierre was killed in 1906 after stepping in front of a horse-drawn carriage, leaving Marie alone to raise their two young girls and to carry on their shared legacy. She won her second Nobel Prize in chemistry in 1911 for her discovery of radium and polonium. After a lifetime dedicated to scientific discovery that led to breakthroughs in modern medicine, especially in oncology, Mme. Curie died of complications caused by prolonged exposure to radiation (Biography.com, 2016).

Our present-day role models have been just as pioneering.

Dr. Patricia Goldman-Rakic, who died in 2003, was a renowned neuroscientist who was the first researcher to fully chart the frontal lobe of the brain, which controls personality, reasoning, planning, insight, and other high-order cognitive functions. Her research contributed immensely to the scientific community's understanding of both Alzheimer's and Parkinson's diseases. Dr. Goldman-Rakic literally took on the philosophical question, "How does the brain create thought?" (McFadden, 2003).

Dr. Regina Benjamin was appointed by President Barack Obama as United States Surgeon General, serving from 2009-2013. Prior to her appointment, Dr. Benjamin served patients at the health clinic she founded in rural Bayou La Batre, Alabama. Despite widespread damage and destruction by Hurricanes George and Katrina, as well as a terrible fire, Dr. Benjamin kept her clinic operating. As U.S. Surgeon General, Dr. Benjamin helped shift the conversation in America from sickness and disease to wellness and prevention through nutrition, physical activity, and stress management (U.S. Department of Health and Human Services, 2016).

Dr. Susan Love, surgeon and breast cancer researcher and advocate, almost went down another path. According to her MAKERS biography, part of a collection of groundbreaking women's stories, as "a good Catholic girl, she joined the convent midway through college, but gave it up after nine months." In 1980 Dr. Love became the first female general surgeon on the staff of Beth Israel Hospital in Boston. Although Dr. Love says she wanted to do all the same "macho" surgeries as the men, she was faced with only female patients, mostly with breast issues. She then found her mission and created the Dr. Susan Love Research Foundation. "I think we can be the generation that stops breast cancer, and that's what drives me," she said in MAKERS (MAKERS, 2016).

It's incredible to reflect on all that women in this country and around the world have accomplished in the field of medicine. Let's keep the momentum going.

Memoirs of a Surgeon's Wife, by Megan Sharma

Let's continue the conversation. And let's be honest about where we are and how we can do better. Let's make sure that in 150 years, people will be astounded by what we've done.

Memoirs of a Surgeon's Wife, by Megan Sharma

WHY DOCTORS LOVE THE VA

The Veterans Administration (VA) has a pretty cool mission statement: "To fulfill President Lincoln's promise 'To care for him who shall have borne the battle, and for his widow, and his orphan' by serving and honoring the men and women who are America's veterans" (U.S. Department of Veterans Affairs, 2016).

Part of this promise includes access to quality medical care at VA hospitals across the country.

During his residency, Arun regularly rotated at the VA, spending months at a time there and countless nights on call.

There was much that Arun absolutely loved about the VA. Of course, it's a privilege to treat and help those who have bravely served our country.

But there are other benefits.

Firstly, as Arun would say, "the customers never complain." Patients at the VA are current or former members of the American military, so it's not surprising that they would exhibit a "yes sir/ma'am" attitude and admiration for authority. This was refreshing for Arun, who didn't always encounter such respectful and positive behavior from his patients.

Part of it may be a generational thing. It's no secret that many people from older generations have more deference for the medical community, than, say, your

Memoirs of a Surgeon's Wife, by Megan Sharma

run-of-the-mill Millennial mommy/blogger who does not believe in vaccinating her children.

It's just different now with technology putting health more firmly into the hands of patients.

There was one thing that Arun found quite insulting about the VA, however. Their computer systems never understood him and never will.

Why?

Because he doesn't have a middle name.

He shall henceforth be known to the VA as Arun X Sharma. I don't see what the big deal is. It sounds like a secret agent code name to me.

Memoirs of a Surgeon's Wife, by Megan Sharma

A DIET SODA ADDICTION: IT COULD BE WORSE

I'm not making light of addiction. Addiction is a serious issue, both for the individuals who suffer from it and for society at large. Fortunately, my husband's addiction during residency only cost an average of $5 per case.

It's sweet. It's bubbly. It's full of chemicals and carcinogens. It is satisfying. It makes you want to eat chips and guacamole. It pops and fizzes when you open it. It is best served over ice. It's...Diet Pepsi!

Yes, Diet Pepsi was a staple in our house for many years. I am convinced there were days that Arun drank way more Diet Pepsi than he ever did good-old-H_2O.

There were a few things that bothered me about the Diet Pepsi:
1. I prefer Diet Coke because it is obviously superior.
2. It was a completely superfluous grocery expense. SHHHHH don't remind me about my $9 organic chocolate bars!
3. Giant 36 packs would take over our already limited kitchen storage space, filling up the fridge, lining the top of the fridge and shelving, and eventually filling up the recycling bags.
4. It made Arun burp and sometimes he would burp in my face and I would nearly vomit.
5. It's just not good for our bodies!

Memoirs of a Surgeon's Wife, by Megan Sharma

So, like any good girlfriend/fiancé/wifey, I encouraged weaning from the Diet Pepsi and we haven't purchased soda regularly in years.

Now we drink Nespresso coffee beverages at home because we're fancy like that. Problem solved.

Memoirs of a Surgeon's Wife, by Megan Sharma

ALWAYS BEHIND

For a doctor, and especially a surgeon, there is no such thing as having your life perfectly together, at any stage in your training or career. The degree of hot messiness varies from lukewarm to white hot disaster, but all doctors fall somewhere on the hot mess scale.

Here's why: doctors are always behind, or feel that they are, in home, work, or (most disturbingly) both.

You don't need to have a family to feel inadequate at home. It happens to single people, too. The goals can be as simple as feeding yourself reasonably healthfully, exercising more than twice a year, keeping your apartment off the show "Hoarders," calling to say hello to your mother often enough that she remembers your birthday, sleeping for a handful of hours, making an appearance at a few social gatherings, and not drinking yourself into oblivion every.single.night. #lifegoals

The tug-of-war between work and home, professional and personal leaves no victors.

When you work too long and too hard, you neglect your family and yourself. When you don't work enough, if "enough" is even definable or attainable, you neglect your clinical and administrative duties and potentially do your patients a disservice. Winning is impossible.

For us, this scenario played out in residency and fellowship, and it happens today in Arun's role as an attending physician. With the demands put on my husband every day, it's not likely to go away any time soon.

Memoirs of a Surgeon's Wife, by Megan Sharma

The amount of time Arun spends responding to emails, phone calls and text messages any time of day or night is absurd. Personal boundaries be damned! The modern physician is always on call.

And the notes. Oh, the notes! Whenever a doctor has any interaction with a patient, from a phone call to a clinic visit to a surgery, they must capture what took place in a written medical note. The note not only serves as part of the patient's permanent medical record, it also protects Arun from liability by clearly outlining how he has treated his patients and what counsel he has offered them.

The result is that Arun must write or review dozens of notes every week. And if he gets behind, he has the billing department, who never work on their weekends, on his butt. They've even started instituting fines to be paid for late notes.

My extreme perfectionist of a husband spends night after night on notes. There isn't a day that goes by that he doesn't have "tons of notes to catch up on."

The pressure is immense and overwhelming. It comes from within, from the boss, from colleagues, from me, from our daughter, and from hospital administrators. If you don't feel the pressure, you're probably dead.

How do we make it work? How do we balance work, family, friends, and a marriage—a near Herculean effort?

I'll tell you our secret. We have learned that time is our most precious commodity. Time together to have fun, relax, and to make memories. Or to just be silly. We are greedy with time and will snatch it up however we can.

Now that we are in a better financial place than we were during residency and fellowship, we hire people to do the things that save our precious family time. We don't mow the lawn; we don't clean the house. We occasionally ask our handy man to do stuff in the attic that we would rather avoid.

I detest meal planning more than attempting to clip my toddler's fingernails, so we started doing meal delivery services that send the recipes and ingredients for gourmet family meals right to our doorstep. A godsend!

Memoirs of a Surgeon's Wife, by Megan Sharma

It's not that we *can't* do these things ourselves. We certainly can. But here's the rub: our free time is quite limited, and we aim to take advantage of it as best we can.

Just because I don't regularly scrub our toilets anymore doesn't make me a despicable person, wife, or mom. I mean, would anyone volunteer to do it for kicks and giggles if they had the choice? I think not.

We let the little things go and say "no" when it's just too much. We take time to have fun together, not just to run errands. We go to the water park or ride the train at the mall just for the heck of it.

Now that I am no longer a tiny chipped piece of tile in the corporate mosaic, it is easier to keep our household running smoothly. But we are both still knackered (to borrow from British vocabulary) by the end of the day.

When we start to snip at one another in frustration, we remind ourselves that we are on the same team (fantastic advice taken from my parents, who have been married since 1980). We try to avoid resentment by setting reasonable expectations about our schedules and always keeping our communication open.

We go on date nights and do exotic things like glow-in-the-dark mini golf, just the two of us.

We have the travel bug, BAD. Our daughter was raised with it—she's been flying since she was two months old and has probably visited more U.S. states and foreign countries (Ireland, Spain, and Mexico by the age of two) than the average adult.

Most importantly, Arun always says that his family is his number one priority, and he backs it up with action. He sets work aside to spend time with us and to help around the house. This usually results in him working while watching TV in the evenings or staying up too late, but he does it willingly.

I try to be cognizant of when Arun is feeling a high degree of pressure from work and (mostly) happily take on more of the household duties.

We aim for at least one night a week when the two of us do absolutely no work and take a breather together. We compromise. We talk. And we listen. We value what one another are thinking and feeling.

Memoirs of a Surgeon's Wife, by Megan Sharma

We try to see things from the other person's perspective and not judge too harshly.

He thinks: "I've been on my feet all day doing four surgeries. I'm so dehydrated that I have a headache. I've barely eaten anything. One of my patients is not doing well and I am worried. I need to write and sign notes. I have a couple of presentations coming up that I need to prepare for. I need to fit in so many surgeries before we leave for vacation and I don't know how I'm going to do it. I'm ready to be done with call."

She thinks: "I've been running around with our daughter all day. She fell asleep in the car for 20 minutes between playdates and then decided that was a sufficient nap for the day. Our house is a mess—there's Tupperware strewn precariously all over the floor. I haven't been able to shower today. I only wanted to eat lunch in peace for 15 minutes, but I didn't even get to do that. I finally got our daughter to bed and scarfed some dinner leftovers and now I'm cleaning up, working on our upcoming trip planning checklist, checking email, and thinking about the writing I want to do tomorrow. I don't have any energy left. And we still have four loads of laundry to fold."

The universe says: it's a tie.

It's not a perfect system and we'll continue to refine it throughout our lives, but we know that we'll always be in it together, and that is reassurance enough.

Memoirs of a Surgeon's Wife, by Megan Sharma

WHEN THE LIGHT AT THE END OF THE TUNNEL COMES INTO VIEW

Six years of residency can feel like sixty. But as you draw nearer and nearer to the finish line, things start to improve. Junior residents, take heart!

Senior residents no longer have the burden of weekend call. This is life changing! Weekends away no longer require vacation time. Social gatherings are duly attended. Significant others are kept happy for a few blissful days. Calendars are marked, and appointments are kept.

The ever-present pager isn't going off like the rhythm of a heartbeat, constantly interrupting the big and small moments of everyday life, from grocery shopping to dentist appointments to Netflix-a-thons. That's because (you guessed it) someone more junior is answering the page first. What a relief.

Here's the real kicker: as a chief resident, Arun earned an extra $150 stipend every month for "administrative duties." These duties, mainly on the job leadership and teaching of junior residents, planning the weekly schedule, and kissing up to attendings, amounted to at least 20 hours per week of additional work. Wow, $1.88 per hour! We've reached the big leagues!

Memoirs of a Surgeon's Wife, by Megan Sharma

And then one day every resident or fellow gets their first real job as an attending. Score! Your immediate reaction is, "shopping spree!" And your next thought is "OH-MY-GOD-WHAT-HAVE-I-GOTTEN-MYSELF-INTO-THESE-ARE-MY-PATIENTS-NOW-AND-I-DON'T-WANT-TO-KILL-THEM-AND-I-DON'T-WANT-THEM-TO-SUE-ME-OH-DEAR-LORD-CAN-I-PLEASE-GO-BACK-TO-BEING-A-RESIDENT-NOW???!!!"

There is greater weight on the shoulders of an attending, in many ways. Community and networking obligations, navigating workplace politics, supervising residents, growing a national reputation, and keeping a constant eye on the tenure track. No more "my 30 service hours are up, see ya!"

Then you start thinking about things like what would happen if I was no longer able to do my job? What if I injured my hands or had a stroke? What if I became blind? So, you fork over a good chunk of that hard-earned attending money for disability insurance.

And then there's retirement. You gotta save for retirement. And save enough that you can maintain a reasonable standard of living when you're older.

Oh, wait—you forgot about your children's college funds and the mortgage. And then Uncle Sam takes his hefty cut.

They say, "it gets better." It does. Mostly it gets different. But the grass is always greener, eh?

Memoirs of a Surgeon's Wife, by Megan Sharma

RESIDENCY GRADUATION DAY

Residency graduation day has finally arrived. It almost doesn't seem possible to have made it to this moment after six blood-sweat-and-tears drenched years. Everything is coming up roses today!

It's June 2014. A day very closely resembling summer in Seattle: cornflower blue skies, a pleasant warmth, plenty of passive-aggressive Northwest "You go. No, you go!" traffic. Arun's family has flown in from Philadelphia for the occasion. My family will also be attending the big event, an annual graduation dinner at the University of Washington.

We have attended the graduation event every year since 2008. It's always been to celebrate someone else's accomplishments. Today, my husband is one of the honored guests. It's finally his turn!

As we graciously accepted congratulations galore from family, friends, and colleagues, we couldn't help but smile until our faces ached.

It didn't matter that we had paid $80 per person for the privilege of providing our family with a catered dinner that wouldn't pass muster in any decent Seattle restaurant. It didn't matter that Arun would still be working at full capacity over the next several days, and that we were given only *five days* to move ourselves, at our own expense, across the country before Arun started his new fellowship in Pittsburgh on July 1st. It didn't matter that Arun's residency graduation gift from the university was a beautiful, engraved wooden office chair that couldn't be packed

Memoirs of a Surgeon's Wife, by Megan Sharma

(since our moving pods were already en route to Pittsburgh), and therefore had to be shipped (again, at our expense) to our new home for $300.

We had arrived! And, guess what else? I was pregnant with our daughter, and only our family knew about our baby joy.

As the familiar program unfolded, it felt surreal, exciting, crazy, strange, and exultant.

When I spotted Arun's mentor, I didn't hesitate to give him a genuine hug. He played a role in Arun's success, too.

My heart was literally bursting with pride and an intense sense of a joint accomplishment. Of course, I cried. I laughed as Arun was roasted by the residents. Of course, they proudly displayed a photo of Arun with his mismatched shoes. I took some video. And then we went home, exhausted, and spent the rest of the weekend saying our goodbyes to friends and family and then making final preparations for our move.

Parents and significant others: when your loved one reaches this milestone, I advise you to do everything in your power to be present in person. It makes the day more meaningful and helps everyone understand how they have contributed to making residency graduation a reality.

And don't forget the champagne. Everyone loves champagne (except covertly pregnant ladies). Cake is an acceptable substitute.

Memoirs of a Surgeon's Wife, by Megan Sharma

LONG DAYS, SHORT YEARS

Many wise parents, grandparents, and great grandparents have said, "The days are long, but the years are short." It's a call to appreciate the fleeting moments of life, even when you may feel like you're just slogging through the mud.

Yes, residency can be a mud fest. But it does have its shining moments, as well.

For one, you are still young and often without children to care for (as we were). You can throw a rooftop barbeque or plan a weekend getaway on a whim. You can go to the late-night sushi happy hour. You can invite your friends over and drink vodka without suffering from the worst hangover of your life the next morning.

You are surrounded by friends and colleagues (and their significant others) who are going through the exact same thing as you. You're allowed to bitch and moan as a group on a regular basis. And you are genuinely thrilled when one of you moves up and out after (too many) years of hard work and sacrifice.

Mistakes are allowed—you are still learning. There will always be somebody there with more experience who can help you out of a pickle. Questions are both accepted and encouraged. Once you become an attending, you're the one being asked the questions.

Discounts! You get discounts on training and conferences because you're still a trainee. There is no Starbucks discount, sadly. There should be.

Memoirs of a Surgeon's Wife, by Megan Sharma

Scrubs are acceptable attire for social events. Because everyone expects that you are overtired, overworked, stressed, and constantly sprinting from one engagement to the next, you get a measure of grace for wearing dirty scrubs out to dinner or to that housewarming party. Later, they'll expect you to change and dress appropriately.

The year before you graduate from residency, you get to mercilessly mock your senior residents and attendings at the graduation roast dinner—consequence-free!

There are still "firsts," like your first complex surgery, first day as a senior resident, first time doing it on your own.

Yes, the days are long. Ungodly long. But the years of residency are short in the larger scheme of things, so don't forget to celebrate the positive moments. If you look for the silver lining, you'll never come up short.

Memoirs of a Surgeon's Wife, by Megan Sharma

AN INTERVIEW WITH THE GOOD DOCTOR

When I asked Arun if I could interview him, he told me that his last interview had been with "GQ," so he was ready. After I stopped laughing and he stopped pouting over my feigned mockery, we sat down for a chat.

MS: Hello, husband.

AS: Hi, wife. Have you heard about my latest book? It's called "Memoirs of a Surgeon's Wife's Husband."

MS: Wow, that is an impressive title and not redundant at all. I am so proud of you! Ok, let's get started.

MS: What is it like to be a surgeon?

AS: It's one of the most rewarding things that I could imagine doing. I have the opportunity to help people in some of their times of greatest need and often the highs and lows of their lives. That's what separates it from many other professions in the sense that it's not just a job, it's a real person who I'm trying to help. I'm very honored to have that opportunity because people literally put their lives in my hands on a daily basis.

MS: What is the best part of your job?

AS: The best part is knowing that I've made a meaningful difference in someone's life. That often means curing them of their head and neck cancer.

Memoirs of a Surgeon's Wife, by Megan Sharma

Another way that I make a meaningful difference is by teaching students and residents who can then go on to impact others in their careers.

MS: What is the worst part of your job?

AS: That would be a tie between dealing with insurance companies and lawyers.

MS: What about people dying?

AS: It's incredibly sad and unfortunate when one of my patients doesn't make it. One of the most difficult things I have to do is talking to the family afterward. I've been surprised in that families are often very grateful for the efforts of the health care team even when their loved one passes away. That said, even though it's a reality of the job, it never gets easier for me.

MS: What was your most embarrassing moment at work?

AS: Wearing a mismatched pair of shoes after being up all night on call.

MS: Eek. That's rough. I remember that day very clearly. I'm glad you've bounced back.

AS: I survived.

MS: What keeps you going and motivated?

AS: My patients often come to me either with a diagnosis of head and neck cancer or I diagnose them as such soon after meeting them. Left untreated, this would often have a very poor prognosis. Knowing that I can make a difference is what keeps me going every day. Seeing patients who have beat their cancer is one of the greatest joys of my job. I've even seen patients and families brought to tears when we have a success. There's no price tag to put on that.

MS: What was your most memorable day on the job?

AS: My first day as an attending physician stands out. At that point, over a decade of training had come to fruition and I was an independent surgeon. Most physicians would recognize that they continue to learn and grow over throughout

Memoirs of a Surgeon's Wife, by Megan Sharma

their career, but starting my career as an academic physician was a memorable day for me.

MS: Now that you have a "real" job, how does it feel?

AS: Exhilarating, yet nerve-wracking. It puts things into a new perspective.

MS: Meaning you're now the boss?

AS: Of course.

MS: What has been your biggest obstacle?

AS: Finding the time to balance everything that is important to me: family and personal life, clinical work and caring for patients, education, and research. In the end, I think I've made it work.

MS: What is your advice to aspiring physicians? Say, a college student?

AS: Learn everything you can. Remember to spend quality time with your family and friends—they are the people who will be with you in the long run. Identify something outside of school or work that you're truly passionate about and stay committed to it. Finally, it's always important to ask yourself if you really want to do this. It can be a hard road at times, but in the end, it's incredibly rewarding.

MS: If you weren't surger-izing, what would you do instead?

AS: I have a list.
1. Spend time with my wife and daughter.
2. Write my book sequel, "Memoirs of a Surgeon's Wife's Stay-at-Home-Husband."
3. Teach young people, whether it's high school students, college students or medical students, a little bit about what I've learned along the way.
4. Research ways to improve quality of life for head and neck cancer patients (the patients I would be surger-izing).

MS: What's it like having a hot and talented wife like me?

AS: It's awesome. I couldn't be luckier. Thanks, Match.com!

MS: Aw, you're cute. I think I'll keep you.

MS: Any last words? Not like you're facing the firing squad or anything. Just to finish off this chapter.

AS: YOLO.

MS: Oh, dear God....

AS: It's always interesting to hear about the paths of various people I work with and to think about my own career trajectory and choices. There's no set formula that works for everyone. However, I feel that I've worked hard and have been blessed by opportunities and excellent mentors along the way. Thinking back five, 10 or 20 years ago, I probably wouldn't expect to be where I am now. That said, I am very satisfied. That's one of the exciting things for me—I'm sure that the coming years will be just as interesting and rewarding.

Memoirs of a Surgeon's Wife, by Megan Sharma

C IS FOR CANCER

Cancer is a murderous monster. Not just because the American Cancer Society estimates it will have killed 1,630 people every day of 2016 in the United States—more than 595,000 people by year's end—but also because it is relentless and will consume anything and everything in its path (American Cancer Society, 2016).

Did you know that cancer, left to its own devices, will literally rot away skin and bone? BONE. Many of Arun's patients have lost portions of their jaw, eyes, nose, tongue, ears, voice boxes, and cheeks to cancer.

Although they may be out of the beauty pageant circuit, this is often what is necessary to save the patient's life via surgery, or what has already happened due to cancer run amuck.

My own dear grandmother, Jacqueline Dodd Pearson, was taken from us too soon by cancer. At age 11, my grandmother was adept at ping pong, jacks, and double dutch. Her ginormous Catholic family of nine children, including her twin brother, Jack, enjoyed gathering around the family radio after dinner every night, knitting or playing games as they listened to the programs. Around this age, she also picked up the habit that would ultimately kill her: smoking.

How did an 11-year-old get her underage hands on cigarettes, you ask? She started smoking cigarette butts from her parents' ashtray down in the basement.

As an adult, Grandma smoked at least a pack a day for several decades, all the while relishing and enjoying life, offering my brother and I the overflowing cookie bucket (a repurposed gallon ice cream container used to store all manner of sugary goodness) as we came sloshing out of their backyard pool for sustenance.

Memoirs of a Surgeon's Wife, by Megan Sharma

First, she battled breast cancer. She lost her hair but not her fighting spirit. After a double mastectomy and several rounds of chemotherapy, she was declared cancer free.

Then she developed lung cancer.

While my memory of the timeline is a bit hazy, I remember this clearly. My mom had flown down to Northern California to be with my grandparents, while my dad stayed with my two brothers and me up in Seattle. We knew that Grandma was sick, and I think that we knew she had cancer again, but we didn't know how serious the situation was.

Until my mom urged my dad to take us out of school immediately and drive down to California—things had gone from bad to worse.

It was an anxiety-filled and tense 14-hour drive. We stopped as little as possible. We were expecting to be greeted by a weaker version of our wonderful Grandma. Instead, we received the devastating news that she had already passed away. We were too late to say a proper goodbye.

Instead of gently clutching Grandma's familiar hand and sitting at her bedside talking and telling our favorite stories, like the one about how her mother schooled the nun who had punished my grandma as a child for getting sick in the classroom, we planned and attended her funeral.

It was an open casket, which was incredibly weird, as Grandma looked like a waxed and rouged version of her former vivacious, passionate self.

We cried and cried and cried. It was the first time I had experienced a significant loss in my life. As I write this, I can't prevent the tears from rolling down.

Grandma was only 71 when she died. I was 16, and I'll never forget it. Seventy-one may not seem "young," but she had such a youthful and exuberant soul that I know she had so much more to give her family and this world.

"Don't we live happy!" she would exclaim joyfully while kicking her feet as we all sat around the kitchen table. She would have cracked jokes with my husband and told him about her childhood dream of becoming a doctor and doted on her great

Memoirs of a Surgeon's Wife, by Megan Sharma

granddaughter like there was no tomorrow. I'm sure we would have seen the reemergence of the cookie bucket, despite any parental protests on my part.

God, I miss her. And, listen, CANCER—YOU SUCK!! You don't belong in this world. And someday we will find a way to banish you forever.

There is hope. Education and prevention of high-risk activities such as smoking and excessive drinking are, of course, part of the picture. Surgical and other oncologic treatment options performed by highly-trained and dedicated physicians and medical teams are also in abundance.

That said, we know our own bodies best. If something doesn't feel quite right, don't hesitate to pay a visit to your doctor.

Time is our most precious possession and if we wait too long to act, we can never get it back.

Memoirs of a Surgeon's Wife, by Megan Sharma

A SIGNIFICANT OTHERS' GUIDE TO SURVIVING RESIDENCY

Scores of books and articles have been written about how to survive residency for the physicians going through it. But here, those suckers are on their OWN. Just kidding.

Really, though, this chapter is for all the significant others out there—the "SOs"—who keep the home fires burning, perhaps while also working full-time and/or raising children, while their loved one treads through the choppy waters of residency, endeavoring to keep from drowning.

To be honest with you, when I met Arun, I didn't think twice about how his career might impact our relationship and our future. We fell in love and nothing else mattered. I was a bit naïve.

Of course, reality did creep into our blissful honeymoon period and there were days that I didn't think I could make it through. Would medicine always come first? Would our lives ever be our own? It sounds ridiculous for me to be complaining about how much *he* was working, I know. But it was hard on both of us when Arun was always (literally, always) studying, checking lab work, writing notes, reading journal articles, preparing presentations, dictating, on call, doing research, and at the hospital.

Memoirs of a Surgeon's Wife, by Megan Sharma

Somebody had to do laundry, clean the condo, buy groceries, cook food, maintain relationships with friends and family, plan for holidays, pay bills, and open the bottles of wine, did they not?

My advice can be applied to anyone with a demanding job or training program, not just to surgical residents and their SOs.

Here's what I've learned coming from the other side of my husband's seven years of training (post medical school).

1. **Don't forget about your own life**. You had a life before you met your SO, and that should not be cast aside simply because you are now part of a pair. When your SO is working-working-working-working-WORKING, you'll need friends and family to hang out with, unless you want to be stuck in front of the TV alone, constantly checking the clock. Keep your weekly brunch date with girlfriends, don't blow off your tennis buddy, have your boys' night out. It's healthy and much more interesting to have hobbies and interests aside from your SO. And if you can, find other SOs in your position to commiserate with. Nobody can understand what you're going through like they can!

2. **Divide the labor**. Just because one person works way more than the other doesn't mean they're off the hook for household duties. When you're living together, it's only fair to have an open conversation about how to "adult" together. Perhaps you love Excel and budgets and your SO prefers to do the cooking. Awesome! But neither of you like to clean the toilets. Then you can alternate, or hire someone to do it, if you can afford to. It's important to be realistic, to give your partner the benefit of the doubt, and to not demand a completely even 50-50 split. Don't expect more than is humanly possible and go easy on yourselves for what you cannot do.

3. **Keep talking to one another**. It is so crucially important in any relationship to maintain open communication. Be honest with your SO about your personal ambitions, career aspirations, family dreams, and the future you want to build together. Throughout Arun's residency, we had many talks about what he might like to specialize in and the lifestyle that would accompany that specialty. There was one sub-specialty he/we chose to avoid because of its demands: 15+ hour surgeries and 24/7 on call surveillance post-surgery. No, thanks. We knew we would eventually want

Memoirs of a Surgeon's Wife, by Megan Sharma

to start a family and we thought carefully about how his career (and mine) could support that. My writing dreams have evolved, as well. I went from years of corporate communications and marketing to writing books, and Arun has always enthusiastically supported me. There are numerous decisions to be made throughout medical training, from where you will live to how much money you want to make to private practice or academic medicine. It's essential to approach these decisions as a team.

4. **Have FUN together!** When you and your SO are stressed, fighting and nit picking can be common. I highly recommend taking every opportunity to enjoy life together and to seize the moment. Did your SO get off work early? Take a walk and grab some dinner! Not on call this weekend? Take that little day trip to wine country you've been talking about for ages. Treasure and guard these fun and adventurous times together. These are the moments that help you get through the tougher times.

5. **Take it one day at a time.** Certain residency rotations (usually lasting three months each) are more challenging than others. Mentally prepare yourself for this and remember that all the years of training are broken down into much smaller chunks of time. Celebrate the smaller milestones along the way, like the day your SO is no longer an intern, or is finally known as a senior resident.

6. **Plan vacations together.** Getting away from it all is so necessary when you and/or your SO work 80+ hours per week. The goal is to have something to look forward to when you're dredged in the muck and mire, and to have heartwarming memories when you return to your daily lives. Go on at least one week-long vacation every year and take long weekends when you can.

7. **Choose not to be resentful.** When your SO is a surgical resident, shit happens. There are birthday parties missed, anniversary dinners postponed, and outings with friends attended solo. The reality is that when a patient needs your SO, he/she has a moral obligation to help them. Plus, it's their job. We can choose to be bitter and grumble interminably about how our SO missed this and that. Or we can try to be flexible and grateful for the time we do have together. I suggest the latter.

8. **Invest in the now.** If you spent all your time waiting and wishing for your SO's training to be over, you'd be missing a huge

opportunity. Life doesn't wait. You can't get that time back, no matter how much you may want to. Is your SO working on Christmas day? Celebrate on the 26th, who cares? Invest in both your career and your relationships right now, rather than just one or the other. They are not mutually exclusive.

9. **Be proud of yourself, too.** Even if you're not the one doing the "doctoring," you have a lot to be proud of. Your loved one couldn't do it without you. From emotional support to chocolate chip cookies to acting as a bonafide sugar mama/daddy during the training years, your contribution is real and it is meaningful.

10. **Keep your eye on the prize.** Remember that it won't always be like this. There will come a day when your SO is the boss and has more control over his/her schedule. There will come a day when your SO doesn't fall asleep every night with his/her face buried in a textbook. And there will come a day when it will be worth all the sacrifices you've both made. I promise!

Memoirs of a Surgeon's Wife, by Megan Sharma

PART 4: LIFE BEYOND RESIDENCY

❖ ❖ ❖ ❖ ❖

Memoirs of a Surgeon's Wife, by Megan Sharma

THE FELLOWSHIP BABY BOOM

Couples often try to time the conception and birth of their babies juuuusssttt right, and we are no different. Teachers aim for a summer birth, and surgical residents aim for the conclusion of residency. For us, as for many of our friends, that was the fellowship year.

It just wasn't practical to start a family during the insanity that was Arun's residency. His 80+ hour workweeks, endless late-night pages and inability to exact any measure of control over his schedule made it a no-go. Plus, we had less than 700 square feet between us and zero spare inches of closet space.

Our lives were chaotic when we first started "trying." Arun was a few months away from finishing residency and we were living in Seattle. I was working hard as ever as a Communications Manager for a bustling IT consulting firm.

We decided to put our condo on the market, knowing that we would be moving to Pittsburgh for Arun's fellowship year, starting July 1, 2014. That meant a massive Goodwill purging, renting an additional storage unit in our building to store boxes that we had pre-packed, staging the condo ourselves, and preparing for dozens of walk-throughs at a moment's notice. Not to mention the back-and-forth with U-Haul customer service for our cross-country move via pod. Nightmare. I don't suggest it!

When the condo sold within about two weeks (thank you, cash buyer!) we were presented with a brand-new challenge: where on earth were we going to live for the next two months?

We didn't have much time to think about it. The closing was scheduled two weeks later and then we had to be out of there!

Memoirs of a Surgeon's Wife, by Megan Sharma

I basically called my mom one day and said, "We are moving in. How is this weekend?" Thankfully, my parents live about 25 miles outside of Seattle, a doable commute. And they were okay with us casually taking over their home for two months while we rode out the rest of residency. They even gave us their bedroom, so we'd have more space and privacy. Parents, right? So sweet.

Shortly after moving back in with my parents (the definition of cool) I learned I was pregnant. Taking two naps a day and not eating much definitely did not fool my mom, who straight up asked me if I was preggo one day. I had been planning to tell her a few days later, so I shrugged it off. We made the announcement on the day we loaded up a bunch of our stuff into a local U-Haul storage unit. That got me out of the heavy lifting.

Once we landed in Pittsburgh, we were confronted with the realities of moving cross-country in only a few days, my continual state of pregnancy, and preparing for Arun to start a new job. Luckily, I could continue my job virtually from Pennsylvania, which eased the transition.

Let's just say that we lived in the land of boxes for quite some time.

Despite the crazy, the timing was good. As close to perfect as it gets. We now had two bedrooms, two bathrooms and 1400 square feet to ourselves. Arun's job was much more predictable, and he worked fewer hours than in residency. I had the flexibility to work from home when I needed it the most, which was helpful, since I was nauseous 24/7 for the first 15 weeks of my pregnancy and kept crackers at the bedside.

Arun's program director in Pittsburgh claimed that there must be something in the water, because all the fellows had young kids or babies on the way.

What he didn't know was that water had absolutely nothing to do with it. The end of residency is the beginning of the baby boom.

Memoirs of a Surgeon's Wife, by Megan Sharma

TALES FROM THE PREGNANCY CRYPT

While writing this book, I experienced the effervescent miracle that is pregnancy. Every day was filled with wonder and new horrors alike.

Let me share a few examples:

<u>The fat lip</u>
One morning (12 weeks and a few days along) I suddenly started gagging and feeling very nauseous (ok, this happened several times a day), but this time I felt all watery and near pukey.

I tried eating a saltine, my usual lifeline. No use. I realized I was going to puke, but too late.

I sprinted to the bathroom and in the process of desperately trying to lift the toilet seat to hit my target, I smashed myself in the face with it before vomiting.

When I looked in the mirror, I already had a fat and semi-bloody lip. I sat icing my lip with breakfast.

Pregnancy is the best!

<u>Daily Realities and other Musings</u>
- The morning "Metamucil cocktail"—skip it and you will pay dearly
- Eating saltine crackers in bed (yes, crumbs are a problem)

Memoirs of a Surgeon's Wife, by Megan Sharma

- Why does everyone choose the exact time that you are pregnant to ask about your child bearing status or plans? (before you are ready to tell them the news)
- I never knew that one day I would pin all my hopes on prune juice. PRUNE JUICE!
- Your attachment to your body pillow becomes an obsession. Results: semi-comfortable sleep and the ultimate cock-block. Sorry, husband.
- Knowing the size of your baby compared to small fruits is a real thrill
- Your urine becomes exceptionally popular with doctors
- Being pregnant and ladylike do not go hand in hand: random burping and farting, sudden GI distress, tantrums over hunger, and crying outbursts are the norm
- The sensation of hunger is replaced exclusively with nausea for the first trimester
- The fire of 10,000 dragons in my chest (constant heartburn!)
- Testing the structural integrity of my winter jackets while eight months pregnant in a sub-zero Pittsburgh winter
- The last month of pregnancy feels like "Groundhog Day" – and not on a day that you deliver your baby. On a day that you feel like a gym full of basketballs all rolled into one giant rubber sphere. One that can barely get out of bed.

I can't complain about pregnancy too much, now that we have our beautiful daughter. Plus, someday she, too will understand these joys.

Good luck with that, little one!

Memoirs of a Surgeon's Wife, by Megan Sharma

THE DAY I BECAME A MOM

January in Pittsburgh, Pennsylvania. Arun and I were spending his fellowship year in Pittsburgh so that he could learn head and neck cancer surgery from the best at the University of Pittsburgh Medical Center (UPMC). The winter was excessively frigid, with numerous days in single or even negative digit temperatures.

I was 39 weeks pregnant, and SO ready to have this baby. It had become a momentous challenge to simply roll over in bed, or to get in and out of bed. I felt enormous and uncomfortable. I had planned to work right up until the delivery (thankfully, I was working from home), which was way tougher than I had imagined it would be. I'd been having those cruel Braxton Hicks contractions off and on for a week, getting excited every time, thinking that it was "time," until the faux contractions would abruptly stop.

On Thursday, January 15th, I had an evening appointment with the OB. She could not tell for sure the position of the baby (facing head down or not), so she recommended that we get an ultrasound to check it out. The following day, Friday, January 16th, Arun was able to take the day off to go with me to my appointment.

We decided to enjoy a special lunch together, first. We went to the Strip District, which is like Pike Place Market in Seattle, and had a yummy lunch at a Caribbean place called Kaya. Mahi mahi sandwiches, mmmm! Then Arun treated me to some gourmet chocolate at my favorite chocolate shop, and we headed to Magee Women's Hospital for our appointment.

The ultrasound technician had two pieces of news: first, our baby was in the perfect birthing position, head down. And then this: I had low amniotic fluid. The

Memoirs of a Surgeon's Wife, by Megan Sharma

tech sent us up to triage and warned us that they would probably admit me, and that I would likely be having a baby tonight. WHOA!

Of course, we had prepared for this moment, but we had not anticipated how it would come about. Our labor and delivery bags were packed with all the necessities and were sitting uselessly at home. We had nothing with us but the clothes on our backs. (Arun went home later for the bags, only a mile away).

We rode the elevator up to the triage level and checked in. Soon, we were occupying a teeny little triage room. I had to put on a hospital gown. I had an IV placed for the first time ever. Mostly, we waited. Nurses came and went. The hospital was busy that night, and they wouldn't usher me into a plush and spacious birthing suite until there was a free bed, and I was actively in labor.

Our OB, Dr. Hoca, gave us more bad news: I was zero percent dilated, zero percent effaced (meaning: no progress in labor whatsoever). We had a choice to make, thanks to the low amniotic fluid: go ahead with a C-section, or chance it with labor by being induced.

It seemed like an impossible decision, and it was one that I immediately cried over. There was no guarantee that I would have a short labor after being induced. I might labor for 20+ hours and then still require surgery. That terrified me more than anything.

In the end, we decided to give Jasmine the chance to come out on her own time, and so I was induced. By this point, we had let our families know that the birth was on the horizon. They were thrilled!

So, Arun and I watched reruns of "Modern Family" on the hospital TV while waiting for labor to begin.

The "bed" was so uncomfortable – it was more like a wheeled apparatus with gym wrestling mats on top – not a real mattress. Thankfully, our nurse was very kind and got me an actual hospital bed. Bless her heart!

All in all, we were in the little triage room for 6-7 hours before a bed in a labor and delivery room became available. Just before that, I had my first contraction. Suddenly, I felt a searing, knife like pain in my hip area. I went from zero to 200, because I had been induced.

Memoirs of a Surgeon's Wife, by Megan Sharma

The contractions started coming more regularly, but still seemed a little random. We tried to settle into the labor and delivery room. Arun put on some music and rubbed my back. Unfortunately, the pain was just too forceful for any of the techniques we learned in childbirth classes to work!

I asked for an epidural, and the anesthesiologist came within minutes to help. It was frightening, but it didn't hurt. I concentrated on following the anesthesiologist's instructions, breathing correctly, and bending my spine just as she had asked. After she injected the medicine, the anesthesiologist checked my degree of numbness.

All the while, I was having extremely painful contractions. I was on my side with monitors on the baby. The nurse wanted me to keep my legs straight, but that felt impossible, since the pain made me want to curl up into a ball. So, they placed an internal monitor.

Suddenly, everyone started chattering at once and I heard a lot of beeping, it must have been on the monitors. I was in a bit of a daze. My lower body was starting to go numb. They had me get on my hands and knees to relieve pressure on the baby. It didn't work.

Before I knew what was happening, they were rolling me out of the birthing suite and to the operating room. I was terrified and started crying. I didn't know if Arun was with me or not, I was still on my hands and knees and looking down at the bed under me.

We arrived in the operating room. It was like laying directly underneath the lights at a baseball stadium – excessively bright, shockingly white. There were people in scrubs all around and a flurry of activity. By then my legs felt like cement blocks. I couldn't move. So, they rolled me onto the operating table. The anesthesiologist checked to make sure I was sufficiently numb for surgery.

I repeatedly asked where Arun was, since he wasn't there. No one bothered to answer me. It seemed like ages had passed. I was on the operating table, but surgery hadn't yet started. Dr. Hoca told me that the baby was safe now, but that it was likely she wouldn't be able to tolerate the contractions much longer. She recommended a C-section, and I agreed. I wanted Jasmine to be safe.

Finally, Arun came into the operating room in a bunny suit. I was so relieved to see him. They had left him confused and alone in the delivery suite. Some

Memoirs of a Surgeon's Wife, by Megan Sharma

of the scariest moments of his life, he said. He was distraught and wanted to be with the baby and me. There was nothing I wanted more in that moment than to hold his hand, and I was so grateful that he was there.

They started the surgery. It was very strange – I could hear everyone talking, the instruments clanging, and could see people near my head, but obviously, there was a sheet blocking my lower body (thank god!). The creepiest thing was feeling my uterus being jerked around, at first. It didn't hurt, it was just odd, like when you're having dental work done with Novocain.

Eventually, I became so numb that I couldn't feel anything. I was naked and absolutely freezing and shivering uncontrollably. My teeth were chattering. I think I was probably in shock. I just kept waiting and waiting for them to hold Jasmine up. I continually prayed that the surgery would go well, and that Jasmine would be healthy.

Finally, after eons, it sounded like they were about to deliver the baby. And then: a miracle. Jasmine was here! It was 1:52 a.m. on January 17, 2015. They held her up above the sheet so that we could see her. Arun, full of emotion with tears in his eyes, exclaimed, "That's our daughter!" We were both overwhelmed with joy and could not wait to hold her.

Jasmine had a strong, clear cry right from the beginning. That was a great sign. She had an Apgar score of 9/10, which is excellent. Arun got to hold her – he was instantly in love. I got to kiss her and snuggle her against my face while the surgeons sewed me up. It was incredible.

Eventually, we went back to a hospital room to recover. I snuggled our little love and breast fed her for the first time. I had never felt such joy, and neither had Arun. It was simply amazing.

Over the next few days, we became a family. We'll always treasure that time we had together, and Arun's three weeks of paternity leave. Arun said it was like our honeymoon: he had never been happier. Neither had I.

Jasmine had completed our world.

Memoirs of a Surgeon's Wife, by Megan Sharma

WHAT IS A PARENT?

It's interesting to realize that the word "parent" is multidimensional, just like the people it describes. In simple terms, a parent is both a noun (person, place or thing) and a verb (an action, state or occurrence). Don't worry, it gets better.

As a noun, it's the people who brought a precious baby into the world, or who adopted him/her as their own. The people who are responsible for that child's well-being. The people who proudly answer the call for "mama" or "dada" at 3:34 a.m. (and then again two hours later).

But, as with so many things in life, being a parent is much more about action. I'm verb-ing from sunrise to sunset as a mom. And my husband is just as verb-a-licious when he's not working his tail off.

What does it look like?

It's putting down your phone and sharing a chuckle with your baby instead of checking your latest text message.

It's meticulously combing the depths of the high chair seat for the latest food morsels: avocado, tofu, broccoli, scrambled eggs, peaches, and the like. And doing this three times a day.

It's reading "Llama Llama Red Pajama" when you can barely keep your own eyes open.

It's spending hours and hours comparing car seat ratings on Consumer Reports and Amazon until you find the perfect one that costs more than $300, just your luck.

Memoirs of a Surgeon's Wife, by Megan Sharma

It's taking her on her very first "choo choo" ride and loving every minute.

It's insisting on socks, even when she just pulls them off three seconds later.

It's celebrating things like digestive regularity. Yes, poop! It's gross!

It's planning for the future, both emotionally and financially.

It's visiting a play place called Ergadoozy and hurting your back while leaning awkwardly over the plastic slide, so that your baby doesn't fall out of the slide structure.

It's all these things, big and small, day in and day out. I can't wait to see what comes next.

Memoirs of a Surgeon's Wife, by Megan Sharma

THE DAWN OF A NEW ERA: B.B. AND A.B.

It was a 6th-century nomadic monk named Dionysius Exiguus who first introduced the world to the concept of quantifying time based on a significant historical event. Dionysius thought the incarnation of Jesus Christ ought to mark the past and present. Hence, the labels, "Before Christ" (B.C.) and "After Death" (A.D.). We are all familiar with these.

For new parents, however, there is only B.B. and A.B.: Before Baby and After Baby.

BB: Coming up with a super book chapter idea and writing it immediately.
AB: Coming up with a super book chapter idea and writing it five months later.

BB: Dreaming of owning a kayak and taking serene morning paddles on the lake.
AB: Splashing around the baby pool and bathtub until she's old enough to swim.

BB: Imagined traveling to Europe with a baby wouldn't be *that* different from previous adventures.
AB: Was I temporarily insane?? I can't even make it to the mailbox on most days!

BB: Phone camera reel includes sappy pics with the hubby, vistas from exotic vacations and delectable foodie treats.
AB: All baby, all the time! And sometimes comparison shopping photos of cribs.

BB: I'm free as a bird! Sure, let's go see a movie. Preferably in a theater that serves martinis.

Memoirs of a Surgeon's Wife, by Megan Sharma

AB: On Demand movies, you have saved our lives.

BB: Used the crock pot only in winter, perhaps a couple of times a year.
AB: A critical tool for our family's survival. Low and slow, baby!

BB: Online shopping for pumps and blazers.
AB: Online shopping for Pampers and bottles.

BB: Schedule as accurate as accurate can be. Thank you, Outlook.
AB: I don't make the schedule. See: the BOSS (baby).

BB: Worrying about spilling Malbec on my new blouse.
AB: Specifically purchasing clothing that will hide inevitable baby slobber and whatnot. Please don't ask me to elaborate on the whatnot.

BB: I can pretty much do whatever I want, whenever I want to do it.
AB: I can't do anything within any reasonable amount of time, but I do have this beautiful, perfect baby to keep me entertained in the meantime.

BB: Life is grand.
AB: Life is grand, hilarious, unpredictable, and oh-so-sweet.

And then, of course, there is the next era: Before Teen and After Teen. More on that in a decade.

Memoirs of a Surgeon's Wife, by Megan Sharma

A BRAND-NEW DAY

Today is tough. I'm not a puddle of tears crumpled on the floor like I expected to be, thankfully. But there is stomach churning. There is stinging guilt. And, oh, there is worry.

Our beautiful almost-16-month-old daughter, Jasmine, started part-time day care today (in May 2016).

It's not like we didn't know this was coming. We have planned it for months. I spent the last five mornings visiting the center with Jasmine to help her ease in.

We have no complaints about the center—the teachers are wonderful and educated in early childhood development, the children are happy and engaged, and the atmosphere is transparent and welcoming. But it's not the same as home and it never will be.

Last night when I should have been sleeping soundly after a super indulgent homemade Mother's Day meal of filet mignon with bacon cream sauce, garlic mashed potatoes, supersized prawns, roasted peppers, and New York style cheesecake (plus a few glasses of merlot), I felt physically ill at the thought of leaving Jasmine, even for a few hours.

I'm not a martyr, nor do I want to be. The truth is that I want what's best for Jas, and for our family. That doesn't make it easy. At least not right now.

What's best for Jas right now is to continue learning and growing and to be around other children. What's best for me right now is to have some time during the workweek to myself, and, most importantly, to sit down and finish writing this very

Memoirs of a Surgeon's Wife, by Megan Sharma

book. And what's best for my husband is for his two girls to be happy, so that he can also be happy.

I cannot wait to be able to tell Jasmine that I am a published author. That she inspired me and inspires me every day to be a better mommy/wife/daughter/sister/friend/neighbor. If I don't reach for my dreams, how will she know that she can do the same?

It sounds like her first day at the center went smoothly, for which I am grateful. Of course, I shouldn't be surprised by her braveness. This is a kid who ran straight into the ocean (on her first encounter) without a second thought.

Did you know that babies need at least four hugs a day for mere *survival*, and many more to thrive? If that's the case, then how many hugs do mommies and daddies need? Infinity. Infinity hugs and kisses.

Even these few hours away from Jas (only about five, now!) have shown me that as much as she needs and depends on me, I also need her. I need her toothy smile. I need to hear her giggle with glee when we do flips on the living room couch. I need to chase her around the kitchen and then snatch her up in my arms.

Our family is starting a new journey. There will be changes. There will be challenges. But there will always be hope and a whole lot of love.

Memoirs of a Surgeon's Wife, by Megan Sharma

WHAT I NEVER EXPECTED ABOUT MIDWEST LIVING

I've been a West Coast girl my entire life, until the year 2014.

I was born in Northern California and spent my childhood in endless golden sunshine, heavily chlorinated backyard pools, seething Sacramento heat, and Santa Cruz surf. Until my parents "made" us move to Washington state right before my 13th birthday. Cue me insisting to friends and family that *they* were moving, but *I* wasn't moving. Mature.

From ages 13 to 30, I lived in and around Seattle. Since I remembered both the pink toe truck (yes, a tow truck outfitted with a giant pink toe) on Mercer and the day the Kingdome was demolished, I could call myself a genuine Seattleite. It took me a few years to truly appreciate the Evergreen State, but, let me tell you: it is a magical place. Natural beauty is abundant (Ocean! Two mountain ranges! One giant active volcano! Forestry! Lakes! Rivers!), and so is super fresh sashimi and other essentials. No wonder the real estate market is skyrocketing.

All this to say, I never imagined myself living anywhere else. My entire extended family on my dad's side lives in Silicon Valley, and my immediate family lives in the Seattle area. Nevertheless, I did move away. I left that West Coast that I love so dearly. I left it for the man I love more than words can convey: my husband.

First, we lived in Pittsburgh for a year. We knew it would be temporary, so we rented an apartment with twice the square footage of our Seattle condo, for the

Memoirs of a Surgeon's Wife, by Megan Sharma

same price as our previous mortgage. That was a good introduction to housing markets outside of the West Coast!

Then came the biggest change of all: we moved to the Midwest. For my husband's dream job. For good.

If someone had told me five years ago that I would be a permanent resident of Illinois, I would have laughed it up. And yet, here we are, making a life for ourselves and for our daughter among the cornfields in the Land of Lincoln.

No offense to my fellow Midwesterners, newbies and lifers alike, but there was one thing I never expected about Midwest living: to like it!

Yes, busy downtown streets and million-dollar rooftop views have been replaced with extra wide highways and sprawling suburbia, but that's okay!

The living is easy.

There is no traffic. Seriously. I can get from one side of town to the other in 15 minutes, regardless of the time of day. No more planning my day/evening based on traffic patterns.

The people are nice. Not fake Seattle nice, but genuinely kind.

On our first few days here, we had rented a Suburban (I know, right? Way to blend in). My husband was about to unload groceries out of this behemoth of a vehicle, when a six pack of Blue Moon came crashing down out of the trunk and all over our driveway. It was a mess of epic proportions, since broken glass, beer, and 90+ degree weather were involved. We didn't even have a broom, a hose, or a bucket to our name.

One of our neighbors witnessed the catastrophe and immediately came over to help. We ended up taking him up on his broom/bucket loaner offer. Then he asked us if we like pulled pork. We are people who say yes to pulled pork. The next day, his wife brought over home smoked pulled pork, coleslaw made from scratch, and sandwich buns. It was such a sweet gesture that made us feel incredibly welcome.

Those aren't the only kind of neighbors we have here. There is wildlife in our backyard. In Seattle, we didn't have a yard. We had an alley, and it wasn't particularly appealing. In our backyard here in Illinois, I have seen all manner of

Memoirs of a Surgeon's Wife, by Megan Sharma

wildlife, including: squirrels, bunnies, cardinals, blue jays, and one brazen beaver that trounces around eating our grass like he owns the place. I assume it's a "he" with commitment issues, since every time I try to get close to him (for a good photograph), he runs away. Hah.

Finally, it's a very family-oriented town. Everyone seems to either be pregnant or have children. Now that we have a family of our own, a feeling of community matters to us.

So, Midwest—I didn't think we would get along, but I am happy to say that we do. Change, like chicken soup, can be good for the soul. But I'm still going to visit Seattle every chance I get.

Memoirs of a Surgeon's Wife, by Megan Sharma

YOU KNOW YOU'RE A MOM OF YOUNG CHILDREN WHEN...

Getting "all dolled up" isn't about beautifying yourself. It means you're having a tea party. With dolls.

You keep kid juice (organic apple juice boxes) and adult juice (Riesling and Merlot) in the house at all times.

You need tummy control...ev-ery-thing.

Only after you've read all the parenting books on the market do you allow yourself to indulge in that tempting NYT Best Seller.

Shoes from your life before kids: heels, a dash of red, a sprinkle of animal print. Shoes from your mom life: they're all flat and hella comfy. That is all.

You wish you had thought of Spanx. You'd totally be rich.

You're tempted to display a few scribbles on construction paper in a museum quality frame.

You are the only person in your household who knows the location of all the food items.

You drink coffee until it's socially acceptable to drink wine.

Memoirs of a Surgeon's Wife, by Megan Sharma

Your idea of a spa treatment is a hot shower—alone.

Just when you don't think your heart could possibly hold any more love, it grows another measure.

If you push your belly out just so, you can look like you're pregnant again. It's a gift.

You enjoy shopping more for children's clothing and accessories than for yourself.

You put on just enough makeup to avoid looking like a zombie. Nothing more, nothing less.

You only have time to catch up with your girlfriends while driving in the car. Thank goodness for Bluetooth systems!

You're a master of the art of the faux shower.

Your parameters for clothing purchases include: will it hide smudges from chocolate chip cookies? Sold.

You're practiced in spelling out buzzwords like "cookie" and "mall" when conversing with your partner.

You listen to Kidz Bop radio when your children are not in the car.

You feel so relaxed when getting your eyebrows waxed that you don't want to get up.

Goldfish crackers are as much a part of your purse as your credit card and driver's license.

Memoirs of a Surgeon's Wife, by Megan Sharma

WHAT WE CAN ALL LEARN FROM AN EPIC TWO-YEAR-OLD TANTRUM

This morning was a real doozy. The kind of morning during which a headache descended on me before I could even change out of my pajamas.

We have been traveling quite a bit in recent weeks with our two-year-old daughter, Jasmine. When we travel, Jasmine tends to become overly attached to us, and it generally takes a few days back in the home routine to recover.

Jasmine woke before 6:00 a.m. in our bed and began wailing for her daddy, who was in the shower. She then edged herself off the bed toward the bathroom, banging on the door to get his attention. Despite my pleas for her to return to bed to snuggle with me, she ignored me, continued crying, and, with gusto, laid herself down on the floor outside the bathroom.

A few minutes after the shower turned off, the door opened, and Arun invited Jasmine in to "help" him get dressed. This was all fine and dandy until Arun had to leave the house to head to work.

She was absolutely inconsolable. Literally screaming at the top of her lungs, tears streaming down her innocent little face. Nothing I said provided any comfort.

Memoirs of a Surgeon's Wife, by Megan Sharma

She wouldn't allow me to hold her. There was nothing I could do but wait out the protest. This meltdown went on for what seemed like an eternity.

Finally, she agreed to come back to bed with me and look at pictures on my phone. Her smile emerged behind her paci. She seemed exhausted.

The crying started up again when I put my phone away, predictably. Somehow, I convinced her to get dressed and got her off to school, thinking, "dear lord, I need a coffee!" A coffee and a stiff drink.

What can we learn from this foray into toddler dramatics?

1. **Stubbornness (sometimes) pays off**. If you set your mind to something and don't take no for an answer, you will sometimes win. Jasmine's stubborn streak won her some extra face time with daddy this morning. But, ultimately, she lost the battle to get him to stay home from work. "The difference between the impossible and the possible lies in a man's determination."—Tommy Lasorda
2. **Logic doesn't always prevail.** There are certain situations in which logic will never overcome. For example, when dealing with a distraught two-year-old. Recognize this scenario and take another tact. "When you can't change the direction of the wind—adjust your sails."—H. Jackson Brown Jr. H.
3. **Accept the things you cannot change.** We would all do well to remember the Serenity Prayer by Reinhold Neibuhr.
4. **The sun will come out tomorrow**. There is always the hope of a better tomorrow, even through the difficulties of the present. "Learn from yesterday, live for today, hope for tomorrow"—Orison Swett Marden.
5. **Never underestimate the power of one's voice**. Toddlers sometimes use it to exasperate their parents into submission. But we adults can use our voices to do great things. "The one thing that you have that nobody else has is you. Your voice, your mind, your story, your vision. So write and draw and build and play and dance and live as only you can."—Neil Gaiman

Memoirs of a Surgeon's Wife, by Megan Sharma

WHY I LOVE MY HUSBAND AND OUR LIFE TOGETHER DEARLY

Wowza. How do you explain a love that you literally could not live without? I will cheat just a touch and borrow some bits and pieces from our wedding ceremony to help paint the picture.

Our officiant, Pat (rest in peace, dear Pat), asked us to write some personal words to one another that would be a surprise and would be read during our ceremony.

Here are the words that Arun chose (as read by our officiant):
"For Arun, marriage is a lifelong commitment to the one you love. It is being able to communicate freely and openly with each other, to relate honestly, to help each other through rough days, as well as to support each other's dreams.

When he thinks of Megan, Arun smiles. She is intelligent and very witty, with an edgy sense of humor. Megan always makes Arun laugh and their verbal sparring livens up their days. Arun values that he and Megan love each other exactly as they are, and they share many of the same interests: exploring Seattle, going on hikes in the nearby area, trying out new restaurants.

Life is more interesting when the two are together because their work, their backgrounds and their personal interests are all different. Arun appreciates how nice it is that each of them brings their own perspectives to daily life.

Memoirs of a Surgeon's Wife, by Megan Sharma

No matter what they are doing, they have a great time together. It isn't the activity or where they are, says Arun, but that they're together – that's what makes all their memories special.

One of those memories was created just about a month after they first began dating. They decided to go to Bainbridge Island for a morning brunch. After eating they explored the island and walked the beach. They saw a couple having their engagement pictures taken. Both laughed, and Megan commented, 'What if that's us one day?'"

These are the words that I chose for our wedding ceremony:
"To me, marriage means choosing a partner to navigate all the ups and downs of life with. It's a mutual commitment to support and uplift one another when the road is rough; to celebrate and to share in the joy when dreams are achieved together; and to always be a best friend and an open book. It also means occasionally sacrificing the last Diet Pepsi or piece of chocolate for your beloved. Yes, Arun, I will do that for you.

Of course, as a little girl, I dreamed about my wedding day and the man I would someday marry. I would surely be married by age 25—well, three years off. I imagined my man to be tall, dark, and handsome—check! But I never could have asked for a more wonderful, smart, giving, and selfless husband-to-be than you. I am a very lucky woman.

Arun, there is so much I love about you. You are the one person who I can never get enough of—the more time I spend with you the more I want to. I am also constantly amazed by the depth of your kindness and compassion, not only with me, but also with both of our families, our friends, and your patients. I appreciate your thirst for adventure and for living life to the fullest. We have so much fun together.

When you called to ask me out for a second date less than 24 hours after our first date, I knew our relationship was different and special from the very beginning. We quickly became inseparable in a way that felt both natural and completely thrilling at the same time. One day a month or two into dating, I felt this strong desire to take care of you—whether you were sick, sleep deprived, hungry, or overworked (usually all the above). That's when I knew I was truly in love."

Have you had your fill of sap and cheese? No? Perfecto! I'll cap off the lovey-dovey-cheese-fest with a poem I wrote a few days before our wedding in May

Memoirs of a Surgeon's Wife, by Megan Sharma

2012. I sprang from bed in the early morning and rushed to write it down fast enough.

I just want to marry you

I just want to marry you...
Because you make me smile
Because you catch me when I fall
Because your laugh is priceless
Because I want to see the world with you
Because we'll still be rollerblading at 80
Because you are my heart
Because you are my soul
Because we belong together

♦ ♦ ♦

Memoirs of a Surgeon's Wife, by Megan Sharma

THE BACK OF BOOK STUFF

❖ ❖ ❖ ❖ ❖

Memoirs of a Surgeon's Wife, by Megan Sharma

ACKNOWLEDGEMENTS

While this is technically my second published book, I will always fondly think of it as my "book baby," because it is the first full-length book I have written.

It wasn't all unicorns and rainbows.

As I mentioned in the introduction, I started writing "Memoirs of a Surgeon's Wife" in October 2013, when inspiration struck me out of the clear blue sky. I was working full-time as a Corporate Communications Manager at the time, dedicating weeknights, weekends and other stolen moments to the penning of this book.

Before I could complete a first draft, life decided to throw pregnancy and then motherhood in my face. Huge blessings that turned my life upside down.

The manuscript sat dormant for a full year, much to my chagrin.

It wasn't until our daughter started part-time day care that I was finally able to turn my attention to writing once again. I was elated to finish the first draft less than six months later.

From there, I spent about a year pursuing traditional publication with some promising leads that never fully developed, until my brilliant husband, Arun, finally convinced me to go for independent publishing.

It's because of Arun that you are reading this book today. I couldn't imagine a more supportive spouse—one who never once doubted me, raised my spirits when I felt like giving up, shared in my victories, and kept me moving forward inch by proverbial inch.

Arun has also dedicated the time to reading the book (several times), ensuring accuracy of the medical scenarios described, sharing personal anecdotes,

Memoirs of a Surgeon's Wife, by Megan Sharma

accompanying me to a week-long writing conference, and a million other kind acts over the nearly five years since the book idea was born.

My husband not only allowed me to follow my authorship dreams, he helped the dream become reality.

Thank you for your tireless cheerleading efforts, my love. I am so grateful and blessed to be your wife.

Our daughter, Jasmine, though still a toddler, never fails to make me smile and even cheers on my writing. Recently, she has asked to look at my book cover design every day, and ooohs and ahhhs over it. It's the cutest thing ever. Thanks for making my heart so happy, Jasmine!

Of course, I have many people to thank for their contributions to "Memoirs of a Surgeon's Wife" and the trajectory of my writing career.

My wonderful parents, Robert and Barbara Marsh, have encouraged my writing since day one. Because of their pride and continual pep talks, I don't even mind editing my mom's annual Christmas letter.

My in-laws, Prabhakar and Jyoti Sharma, have delighted me with their genuine enthusiasm for my writing. I can always count on them to read and then share my latest works with all their friends.

I have three awesome younger brothers: Trevor and Troy Marsh, and my brother-in-law, Amar Sharma. Although I never did get that sister I always wanted, I couldn't ask for a better set of ruffians than you three. Thank you for making me feel good about my writing.

My gratitude goes out to the extended Marsh/Pearson and Sharma/Raizada families, who have faithfully read my blog and taken up the torch for this book. To Mummiji and all my buas, uncles, aunts and cousins from California to New Jersey to New Delhi and beyond, you are loved and appreciated.

For their legacy and love of reading and writing, I must thank my grandparents, Charles and Phyllis Marsh. Though I use a computer and you use a pencil and paper, we share the same passion for the written word, Grandpa!

Memoirs of a Surgeon's Wife, by Megan Sharma

To my best friend, Melinda Beirnes, who set history in motion by accepting my lunch invitation that day in 8th grade, I couldn't have done it without you. You'll always be my sister.

For everything from reading early chapters to testing out titles and marketing campaigns, I thank my college besties: Michelle Nobles, Erica Clingan, Melissa Sawatzky, Kirsten O'Brien and Kiara Buechler. Our hairstyles may have changed since the early 2000s, but our friendships are timeless.

I have my remarkable friend and neighbor Samantha Saini to thank for creating the cover design for "Memoirs of a Surgeon's Wife," and for promoting my writing efforts on her own time. Sam, I couldn't be happier that we bought the house across the street from your family!

To Doctor Eli Goodman, a true modern-day Renaissance man: the foreword you wrote for this book left me speechless, in the best way possible! Thank you for your continual mentorship, super-human connector abilities, and encouragement. It's been my honor learning from you.

To my new friend Hillary LaMontagne, who clearly missed her calling as a copy editor, thank you for reading my book cover-to-cover in record time, and for making editing fun.

Thank you to the mamas of my local MOMS Club for your perpetual optimism and for keeping me sane as I adjusted to a new city and to motherhood.

I appreciate my former Avanade friends and colleagues, especially Francis Delgado, who truly believed in my writing and that I was destined to do great things.

This book would not have been possible without the advice and contributions of several surgeon friends, who, although anonymous, know just how much they rock. Thank you for taking the time to answer my questions, review book chapters, and share your experiences with the world.

Thanks to Elizabeth Watson for her very thorough book editing and insightful feedback. You helped make "Memoirs of a Surgeon's Wife" better.

Last, but absolutely not least, I owe a great debt of gratitude to my VIP Book Launch Team for volunteering to help make the launch of "Memoirs of a Surgeon's

Wife" a great success. I can't thank you enough for generously sharing your time in support of this book.

Lord, I hope I didn't forget anyone. If I did, I will buy you a beer, and then sneakily add you to the roster, because you can do that with self-publishing (WIN!).

My heartfelt thanks to every one of you!

Signing off with a big, fat smile,

Megan

Memoirs of a Surgeon's Wife, by Megan Sharma

ABOUT THE AUTHOR

Megan Sharma is an author and writing professional originally from Seattle and recently transplanted to the Midwest. In 2015, the same year she moved cross-country (again!) and became a mother, Megan traded her 9:00 to 5:00 for calling the shots in her own writing career.

Visit Megan's web site, www.megansharma.com, to check out her books, her blog, The Savvy Surgeon's Wife, and cool freebies for email subscribers.

When she isn't writing (a rare occurrence), Megan enjoys globetrotting with her surgeon hubby and daughter, cooking and eating delicious food, photography, and yelling at pundits on CNN. Follow Megan via @MegganNSharma on Twitter and @authormegansharma on Facebook.

Memoirs of a Surgeon's Wife, by Megan Sharma

OTHER BOOKS BY THIS AUTHOR

Megan Sharma is the author of "100 of Your Toughest Business Emails: Solved: Plug and Play Ideas From a Seasoned Corporate Communications Manager," available for free in all major digital formats, and also available for purchase in paperback on Amazon.

You can find the book on Amazon, Barnes and Noble, Apple iBooks, Kobo, Blio and Smashwords. All Megan's books can be found on her web site at www.megansharma.com.

Book description

Even the savviest office workers struggle with awkward, sticky and downright tricky business emails. How do I politely tell a colleague that their request isn't my job? What do I say when I'm behind schedule or over budget? What if I hate working with that person? "100 of Your Toughest Business Emails: Solved" has all these answers, and more, from an experienced Corporate Communications Manager.

Most business people, aside from executives, don't have the luxury of leaving their most critical business emails in the hands of trained professionals.

What about the rest of us?

In "100 of Your Toughest Business Emails: Solved", author Megan Sharma draws on her years of experience as a professional ghostwriter for a fast-paced IT company to help others who may struggle with word choice in business emails.

Memoirs of a Surgeon's Wife, by Megan Sharma

The language of corporate America is complex and often filled with potential landmines, which Sharma helps readers stealthily avoid.

"100 of Your Toughest Business Emails: Solved" outlines questions to ask yourself before hitting 'Send', and provides concrete examples in six categories:

1. The Work
2. Spill It! (Questions)
3. Survey Says... (Answers or Statements)
4. Co-Workers
5. Gripes (Complaints)
6. All the Feels (Feelings)

Readers need only find the sentiments for what they wish to say and then choose an appropriate alternative from Sharma's curated lists.

For anyone who sends email in our ever-globalizing working world, this is crucial guide.

Future books

Megan Sharma plans to write and publish the following books in the future:

- "The Blessings and Blunders of Parenthood: The Savvy Surgeon's Wife Tells It Like It Is," a humor book on parenting
- "The Diaper Bag Guide to Traveling with Your Baby or Toddler," a helpful how-to guide based on Sharma's dozens of domestic and international travel experiences with her husband and toddler
- A sequel to "100 of Your Toughest Business Emails: Solved" focused on 100 more difficult business conversations
- Children's books
- Whatever floats her boat, honestly. The sky is the limit.

Stay tuned to www.megansharma.com for the latest on new book releases!

Memoirs of a Surgeon's Wife, by Megan Sharma

CONNECT WITH MEGAN SHARMA

Thank you for reading my book! You, dear reader, are why I dreamed of becoming an author.

If you enjoyed this book, I humbly ask for your written review on Amazon and/or Goodreads. We authors appreciate reviews (almost) as much as a strong cup of coffee.

Online, I write and post about love, parenting, writerly pursuits, and this daring adventure we call life.

In addition, I would absolutely love to connect with you. Find me and let's get social!

Twitter: http://twitter.com/MegannSharma

Facebook: http://www.facebook.com/authormegansharma

LinkedIn: http://linkedin.com/in/megansharma/

Pinterest: https://www.pinterest.com/megzsharma/

Amazon:
https://www.amazon.com/MeganSharma/e/B074P7LLGP/ref=dp_byline_cont_ebooks_1

Memoirs of a Surgeon's Wife, by Megan Sharma

Goodreads:
https://www.goodreads.com/author/show/17072208.Megan_Sharma

Blog: http://www.megansharma.com/my-blog

Freebies for email subscribers:
http://www.megansharma.com/freestuff.html

Subscribe to email updates: http://eepurl.com/cliM21

Web site: http://www.megansharma.com/

Email me: megan@megansharma.com

Memoirs of a Surgeon's Wife, by Megan Sharma

BONUS: DON'T LEAVE JUST YET!

I never want my readers to finish a book and go away empty-handed. Just like I always bring something to a party (usually wine, which no one ever complains about).

While I don't have any vino for you, I would like to share an **exclusive preview** of my upcoming humor book, "The Blessings and Blunders of Parenthood: The Savvy Surgeon's Wife Tells It Like It Is."

If you're pregnant, a parent, grandparent, or have ever spent time around kids, you will get a kick out of this book.

To get your FREE sneak peek of "The Blessings and Blunders of Parenthood," visit https://mailchi.mp/c68ca1880a9f/parentingbookpreview and add your name to my weekly email roster.

Okay, now is your cue to exit stage left. You know what to do!

Cheers!

Best,

Megan

REFERENCES

AAMC. (2016, June 11). *2013-2014 Survey of Resident/Fellow Stipends and Benefits Report.* Retrieved from AAMC.org report: https://www.aamc.org/download/359792/data/2013stipendsurveyreportfinal.pdf

AAMC. (2016, June 6). *DISTRIBUTION OF RESIDENTS BY SPECIALTY, 2003 COMPARED TO 2013.* Retrieved from AAMC.org: https://www.aamc.org/download/411784/data/2014_table2.pdf

AAMC. (2016, December 6). *FACTS: Applicants, Matriculants, Enrollment, Graduates, MD/PhD, and Residency Applicants Data.* Retrieved from AAMC.org: https://www.aamc.org/download/321442/data/factstablea1.pdf

AAMC. (2016, March). *Medical Student Education: Debt, Costs, and Loan Repayment Fact Card.* Retrieved from members.aamc.org: https://members.aamc.org/eweb/upload/2016_Debt_Fact_Card.pdf

AAMC. (2016, June 6). *TABLE 4A: DISTRIBUTION OF WOMEN M.D. FACULTY BY DEPARTMENT AND RANK, 2014.* Retrieved from AAMC.org: https://www.aamc.org/download/411788/data/2014_table4a.pdf

AAMC. (2016, June 6). *TABLE 9A: 2013 BENCHMARKING—PERMANENT DIVISION/SECTION CHIEFS AND DEPARTMENT CHAIRS.* Retrieved from AAMC.org: https://www.aamc.org/download/411802/data/2014_table9a.pdf

AAMC. (2016, June 3). *The State of Women in Academic Medicine: The Pipeline and Pathways to Leadership, 2013-2014.* Retrieved from AAMC.org: https://www.aamc.org/members/gwims/statistics/

AAMC. (2017, March). *Applying to Medical School.* Retrieved from students-residents.aamc.org: https://students-residents.aamc.org/applying-medical-school/article/online-practice-mcat-exam/

AAMC. (2017, March). *Applying to Medical School.* Retrieved from students-residents.aamc.org: https://students-residents.aamc.org/applying-medical-school/article/applying-medical-school/

AAMC. (2017, March). *Applying to Medical School with AMCAS.* Retrieved from students-residents.aamc.org: https://students-residents.aamc.org/applying-medical-school/applying-medical-school-process/applying-medical-school-amcas/

AAMC. (2017, March). *Electronic Residency Application System (ERAS) Historical specialty specific data*. Retrieved from www.aamc.org/services/eras: https://www.aamc.org/download/359232/data/all.pdf

AAMC. (2017, March 9). *Fees for ERAS Fellowship Applications*. Retrieved from AAMC.org: https://students-residents.aamc.org/training-residency-fellowship/article/fees-for-eras-fellowship-applications/

AAMC. (2017, March 9). *Fees for ERAS Residency Applications*. Retrieved from AAMC for Students, Applicants and Residents: https://students-residents.aamc.org/attending-medical-school/article/fees-eras-residency-applications/

AAMC. (2017, March). *The MCAT® Essentials for Testing Year 2017*. Retrieved from AAMC.org: https://aamc-orange.global.ssl.fastly.net/production/media/filer_public/86/fc/86fc423b-69c5-4339-839a-91039bf2c2cf/essentials_2017_-_final_01102017.pdf

AAMC. (2017, March). *You can Afford Medical School*. Retrieved from AAMC Students, Applicants and Residents: https://students-residents.aamc.org/choosing-medical-career/article/you-can-afford-medical-school/

ACGME. (2016, March). *Duty Hours*. Retrieved from www.acgme.org: http://www.acgme.org/What-We-Do/Accreditation/Duty-Hours/GraduateMedicalEducation/DutyHours

AMA. (2017, March 9). *State Medical Licensure Requirements and Statistics 2014*. Retrieved from AMA Store: https://commerce.ama-assn.org/store/catalog/productDetail.jsp?product_id=prod2420009&sku_id=sku2420012&navAction=push

AMA Insurance. (2016, September 14). *2014 Work/Life Profiles of Today's U.S. Physician*. Retrieved from AMA Insurance: https://www.amainsure.com/reports/work-life-profiles-of-todays-us-physician.html

American Board of Otolaryngology. (2017, March 9). *Important Dates and Fees*. Retrieved from ABOTO.org: http://www.aboto.org/important-dates-fees.html#qua

American Cancer Society. (2016, October 10). *Cancer Statistics Center*. Retrieved from Cancerstatisticscenter.cancer.org: https://cancerstatisticscenter.cancer.org/?_ga=1.101602374.633201677.1476107913#/

American Foundation for Suicide Prevention. (2016, August 15). *Physician and Medical Student Depression and Suicide Prevention*. Retrieved from afsp.org: https://afsp.org/our-work/education/physician-medical-student-depression-suicide-prevention/

American Medical Association. (2016, June 24). *Here's how many residency programs med students really apply to*. Retrieved from AMA Wire: http://www.ama-assn.org/ama/ama-wire/post/heres-many-residency-programs-students-really-apply

American Medical Association. (2016, October 10). *Women in Medicine Timeline: A Look at Innovators and Leaders.* Retrieved from American Medical Association: http://www.ama-assn.org/ama/pub/about-ama/our-people/member-groups-sections/women-physicians-section/women-medicine-history/women-in-medicine-timeline.page

American Medical Women's Association. (2016, October 10). *Dr. Bertha Van Hoosen.* Retrieved from American Medical Women's Association: https://www.amwa-doc.org/faces/dr-bertha-van-hoosen/

American Red Cross. (2016, October 10). *Founder Clara Barton.* Retrieved from Redcross.org: http://www.redcross.org/about-us/history/clara-barton

Anupam B. Jena, M. P., Olenski, A. R., & Daniel M. Blumenthal, M. M. (2016, September). Sex Differences in Physician Salary in US Public Medical Schools. *JAMA Internal Medicine,* pp. http://jamanetwork.com/journals/jamainternalmedicine/article-abstract/2532788.

Association of American Medical Colleges (AAMC). (2017). *MCAT - The Official Guide to the MCAT® Exam, Fourth Edition.* Retrieved from Publications - AAMC: https://members.aamc.org/eweb/DynamicPage.aspx?Action=Add&ObjectKey From=1A83491A-9853-4C87-86A4-F7D95601C2E2&WebCode=ProdDetailAdd&DoNotSave=yes&ParentObject=Ce ntralizedOrderEntry&ParentDataObject=Invoice%20Detail&ivd_formkey=6 9202792-63d7-4ba2-bf4e-a0da4

Association of American Medical Colleges. (2013). *Medical Student Education: Debt, Costs, and Loan Repayment Fact Card.* Retrieved from AAMC.org: https://www.aamc.org/download/152968/data/debtfactcard.pdf

Atul Gawande, M. M. (2012, May 3). *Two Hundred Years of Surgery.* Retrieved from New England Journal of Medicine: http://www.nejm.org/doi/full/10.1056/NEJMra1202392#t=article

Bellis, M. (2013, October 27). *About.com History of Pagers and Beepers.* Retrieved from About.com: http://inventors.about.com/od/pstartinventions/a/pager.htm

Bellis, M. (2013, October 27). *About.com: Walkie Talkie - Al Gross.* Retrieved from About.com: http://inventors.about.com/library/inventors/bl_walkie_talkie.htm

Benson, N. M., Stickle, T. R., & Raszka, W. V. (2015). Going "Fourth" From Medical School: Fourth-Year Medical Students' Perspectives on the Fourth Year of Medical School. *Academic Medicine: Journal of the Association of American Medical Colleges,* abstract.

Biography.com. (2016, October 10). *Marie Curie Biography.* Retrieved from Biography.com: http://www.biography.com/people/marie-curie-9263538

CareerBuilder. (2016, May 27). *Press release: 51 Percent of Employed 2014 College Grads Are in Jobs That Don't Require a Degree, Finds CareerBuilder Survey.* Retrieved from CareerBuilder: http://www.careerbuilder.com/share/aboutus/pressreleasesdetail.aspx?sd=10%2F9%2F2014&id=pr846&ed=10%2F9%2F2099

CareerBuilder. (2016, May 27). *Press release: CareerBuilder Launches "Find Your Calling" Initiative With Powerful Insights to Help Students and Parents Discover the Right Careers.* Retrieved from CareerBuilder: http://www.careerbuilder.com/share/aboutus/pressreleasesdetail.aspx?sd=10%2f1%2f2015&siteid=cbpr&sc_cmp1=cb_pr915_&id=pr915&ed=12%2f31%2f2015

CareerBuilder. (2016, May 27). *Press release: New CareerBuilder and Emsi Analysis Finds College Degrees Are Not Keeping Up With Demand in Critical Areas.* Retrieved from CareerBuilder: http://www.careerbuilder.com/share/aboutus/pressreleasesdetail.aspx?sd=3%2f3%2f2016&siteid=cbpr&sc_cmp1=cb_pr937_&id=pr937&ed=12%2f31%2f2016

Charles A. Lee, M. (1849, January 23). *Valedictory Address to the Graduating Class of Geneva Medical College at the Public Commencement.* Retrieved from National Library of Medicine: https://www.nlm.nih.gov/exhibition/blackwell/graduation.html

College Board. (2014, February 11). *Trends in Higher Education: Average Estimated Undergraduate Budgets, 2013-14.* Retrieved from Collegeboard.org: http://trends.collegeboard.org/college-pricing/figures-tables/average-estimated-undergraduate-budgets-2013-14

College Board. (2014, February 11). *Trends in Higher Education: Tuition and Fee and Room and Board Charges over Time.* Retrieved from Collegeboard.org: http://trends.collegeboard.org/college-pricing/figures-tables/tuition-and-fee-and-room-and-board-charges-over-time

College Board. (2016). *Trends in College Pricing 2016.* Retrieved from Collegeboard.org: https://trends.collegeboard.org/sites/default/files/2016-trends-college-pricing-web_0.pdf

Dr. Elizabeth Blackwell, D. E. (1860). *Medicine as a profession for women.* Retrieved from National Library of Medicine archives: https://archive.org/details/62630060R.nlm.nih.gov

Forbes. (2016, June 11). *The best places for business and careers: Seattle.* Retrieved from Forbes.com: http://www.forbes.com/places/wa/seattle/

Memoirs of a Surgeon's Wife, by Megan Sharma

Gagné P, M. J. (2011). Psychopathology and suicide among Quebec physicians: a nested case control study. *Depress Res Treat*, 2011:936327.

Herbst, D. A. (2016, October 4). This is the kind of sexism women who want to be doctors deal with in med school. *The Washington Post*, pp. https://www.washingtonpost.com/posteverything/wp/2016/10/04/this-is-the-kind-of-sexism-women-who-want-to-be-doctors-deal-with-in-med-school/?utm_term=.a3d0637c3461.

Johns Hopkins Medicine. (2014, January 31). *About Johns Hopkins Medicine*. Retrieved from Hopkinsmedicine.org: http://www.hopkinsmedicine.org/about/history/history5.html

Justin S. Golub, M., Michael M. Johns, I. M., Paul S. Weiss, M., & Atul K. Ramesh, B. R. (2008). Burnout in Academic Faculty of Otolaryngology—Head and Neck Surgery. *The Laryngoscope*, 1951-1956.

Justin S. Golub, P. S. (2007). Burnout in Residents of Otolaryngology–Head and Neck Surgery: A National Inquiry into the Health of Residency Training. *Academic Medicine*, 596-601.

Kaplan. (2017, March). *MCAT Prep near Seattle, WA 98121*. Retrieved from Kaplan Test Prep: https://www.kaptest.com/MCAT/enroll?zip=98121

Lebowitz, S. (2015, October 24). Here's how the 40-hour workweek became the standard in America. *Business Insider*.

Leslie Kane, M. (2014, March 11). *Employed Doctors Report: Are They Better Off?* Retrieved from Medscape: http://www.medscape.com/features/slideshow/public/employed-doctors#3

Louise B Andrew, M. J. (2016, August 15). *Physician Suicide*. Retrieved from Medscape: http://emedicine.medscape.com/article/806779-overview

MAKERS. (2016, October 10). *Dr. Susan Love: Breast Cancer Pioneer*. Retrieved from MAKERS: http://www.makers.com/dr-susan-love

Maslach, L. C. (1996). *Maslach Burnout Inventory Manual*. Palo Alto: CPP, Inc.

McFadden, R. D. (2003, August 4). Patricia S. Goldman-Rakic, Neuroscientist, Dies at 66. *The New York Times*, pp. http://www.nytimes.com/2003/08/04/nyregion/patricia-s-goldman-rakic-neuroscientist-dies-at-66.html?_r=0.

National Library of Medicine. (2016, Jne 3). *Biography: Dr. Elizabeth Blackwell*. Retrieved from Changing the Face of Medicine: https://www.nlm.nih.gov/changingthefaceofmedicine/physicians/biography_35.html

NRMP. (2016, March 26). *2016 Main Residency Match® By the Numbers*. Retrieved from NRMP.org: http://www.nrmp.org/wp-content/uploads/2016/03/Match-By-the-Numbers.pdf

Numbeo. (2017, March 9). *Cost of Living Comparison between Pittsburgh, PA and Seattle, WA*. Retrieved from Numbeo: https://www.numbeo.com/cost-of-living/compare_cities.jsp?country1=United+States&country2=United+States&city1=Pittsburgh%2C+PA&city2=Seattle%2C+WA

Page, L. (2016, June 15). *Employed Doctors Report 2016: Who's Happier—Employed or Self-employed Doctors?* Retrieved from Medscape: http://www.medscape.com/features/slideshow/public/employed-doctors-2016#page=9

Salary.com. (2016, June 11). *11 Odd Jobs with High Salaries*. Retrieved from Salary.com: http://www.salary.com/11-odd-jobs-with-high-salaries

Seattle.gov. (2016, June 15). *Seattle's Minimum Wage Ordinance went into effect on April 1, 2015*. Retrieved from Seattle.gov: http://www.seattle.gov/laborstandards/ordinances/minimum-wage

Shanafelt TD, B. C. (2011). Special report: suicidal ideation among American surgeons. *Arch Surg.*, 146(1):54–62.

Tait D. Shanafelt, M. G. (2015). Impact of Organizational Leadership on Physician Burnout and Satisfaction. *Mayo Clinic Proceedings*, 432–440.

Tait D. Shanafelt, M. L. (2016). Relationship Between Clerical Burden and Characteristics of the Electronic Environment With Physician Burnout and Professional Satisfaction. *Mayo Clinic Proceedings*, 836–848.

The Osler Institute. (2016, June 29). *Otolaryngology*. Retrieved from Osler.org: https://www.osler.org/main/ent.html

U.S. Department of Health and Human Services. (2016, October 2016). *Regina M. Benjamin (2009-2013)*. Retrieved from Surgeongeneral.gov: http://www.surgeongeneral.gov/about/previous/biobenjamin.html

U.S. Department of Veterans Affairs. (2016, May 25). *About VA*. Retrieved from VA.gov: http://www.va.gov/about_va/

U.S. National Library of Medicine. (2016, October 10). *Biography: Dr. Mary Edwards Walker*. Retrieved from U.S. National Library of Medicine: https://www.nlm.nih.gov/changingthefaceofmedicine/physicians/biography_325.html

U.S. National Library of Medicine. (2016, October 10). *Changing the Face of Medicine*. Retrieved from U.S. National Library of Medicine: https://www.nlm.nih.gov/changingthefaceofmedicine/exhibition/sights_glass.html

U.S. National Library of Medicine. (2016, October 10). *Changing the face of medicine: Dr. Rebecca Lee Crumpler*. Retrieved from U.S. National Library of Medicine: https://www.nlm.nih.gov/changingthefaceofmedicine/physicians/biography_73.html

U.S. National Library of Medicine. (2016, September 26). *History of Medicine: Elizabeth Blackwell*. Retrieved from U.S. National Library of Medicine History of Medicine: https://www.nlm.nih.gov/exhibition/blackwell/admission.html

U.S. National Library of Medicine. (2016, October 10). *The Rosalind Franklin Papers: Biographical Information*. Retrieved from U.S. National Library of Medicine: https://profiles.nlm.nih.gov/ps/retrieve/Narrative/KR/p-nid/183

United States Census Bureau. (2012). *Educational Attainment in the United States: 2012 - Detailed Tables*. Retrieved from Census.gov: http://www.census.gov/hhes/socdemo/education/data/cps/2012/tables.html

US Census Bureau. (2016, June 11). *QuickFacts Seattle, Washington*. Retrieved from Census.gov: http://www.census.gov/quickfacts/table/PST045215/5363000

Washington State Department of Health. (2017, March 9). *Fee Schedule*. Retrieved from DOH.WA.gov: http://www.doh.wa.gov/LicensesPermitsandCertificates/MedicalCommission/MedicalLicensing/Fees

WebMD. (2016, July 25). *Tuberculin Skin Test*. Retrieved from WebMD.com: http://www.webmd.com/a-to-z-guides/tuberculin-skin-tests

WebMD. (2016, July 25). *Understanding Tuberculosis -- the Basics*. Retrieved from WebMD.com: http://www.webmd.com/lung/understanding-tuberculosis-basics

Wible, P. (2014, July 14). *When doctors commit suicide, it's often hushed up*. Retrieved from The Washington Post.com: https://www.washingtonpost.com/national/health-science/when-doctors-commit-suicide-its-often-hushed-up/2014/07/14/d8f6eda8-e0fb-11e3-9743-bb9b59cde7b9_story.html

Wikipedia. (2016, June 3). *History of medicine in the United States*. Retrieved from Wikipedia.org: https://en.wikipedia.org/wiki/History_of_medicine_in_the_United_States

Wikipedia. (2016, May 26). *Public holidays in India*. Retrieved from Wikipedia.org: https://en.wikipedia.org/wiki/Public_holidays_in_India

Made in the USA
Lexington, KY
29 July 2018